Nutrition and Food

Nutrition and Food

By

Luis E. Voyer

Cambridge
Scholars
Publishing

Nutrition and Food

By Luis E. Voyer

This book first published 2022

Cambridge Scholars Publishing

Lady Stephenson Library, Newcastle upon Tyne, NE6 2PA, UK

British Library Cataloguing in Publication Data
A catalogue record for this book is available from the British Library

ISBN (10): 1-5275-8976-5
ISBN (13): 978-1-5275-8976-6

Contents

List of Figures
(See Colour Centrefold)

LIST OF TABLES

ACKNOWLEDGEMENTS

To Pablo H. Voyer, Professor of Graphic Design, Buenos Aires University, Argentina, for guidance and presentation of graphic material.

To Hilda V. Cortal, psychologist, for her contribution from a reader's point of view

To Mrs Mirta Tula, for her culinary recipes.

To Mrs Elanor Harris, for her excellent proofreading

ABBREVIATIONS

AA	arachidonic acid
ADP	adenosine diphosphate
AGEs	advanced glycation end products
AMP	adenosine monophosphate
ATPa	denosine triphosphate
CRP	C-reactive protein
DHA	docosahexanoic acid
EPA	eicosapentaenoic acid
GI	glycemic index
GL	glycemic load
GSH	reduced glutathione
GSSG	oxidized glutathione
HbA_{1c}	glycated haemoglobin
HDL	high-density lipid
HFCS	high fructose corn syrup
HOMA	homeostasis model assessment index
Ig	immunoglobulin
IL 6	Interleukin 6
LDL	low-density lipid
MTHFR	metyltetrahydrofolate reductase
NCEP	National Cholesterol Education Program
NAD	nicotinamide adenine dinucleotide
NADP	nicotinamide adenine dinucleotide phosphate
NAE	net acid excretion
NSAIDs	non-steroid anti-inflammatory drugs
TNFα	tumour necrosis factor-alpha

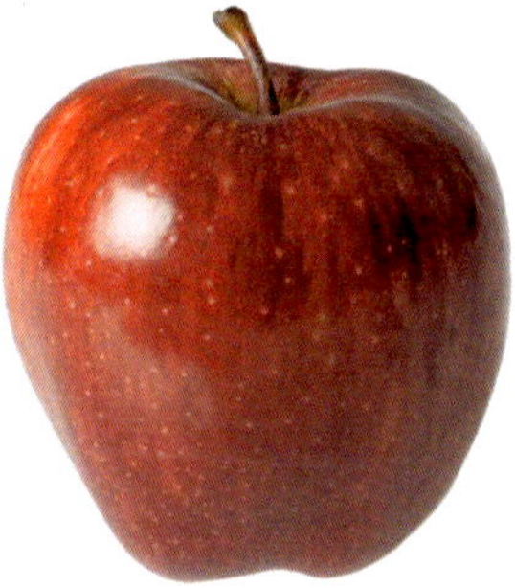

Photo 1-1: Apple

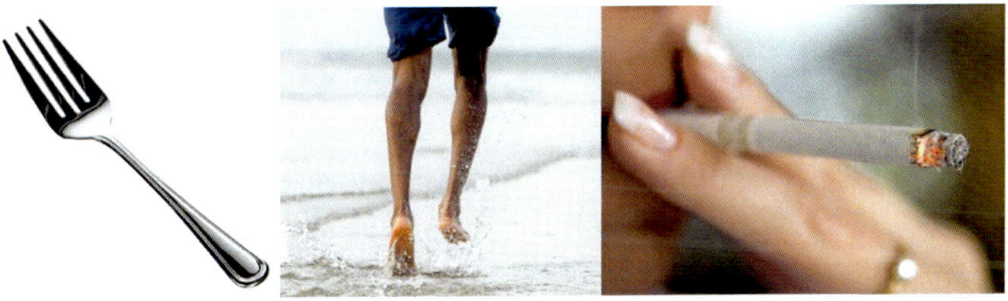

Photo 1-2: Factors that make up health or disease behaviours

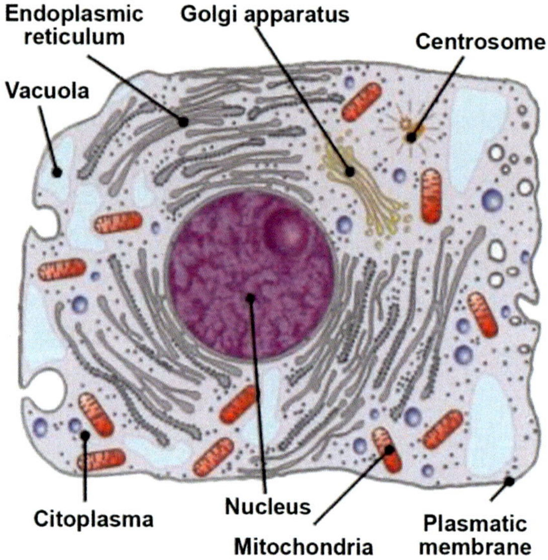

Fig. 1-1: A cell with the nucleus and organelles

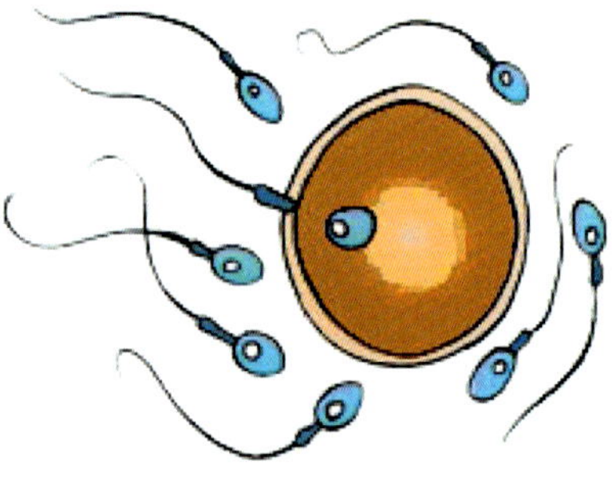

Fig. 1-2: Fecundation

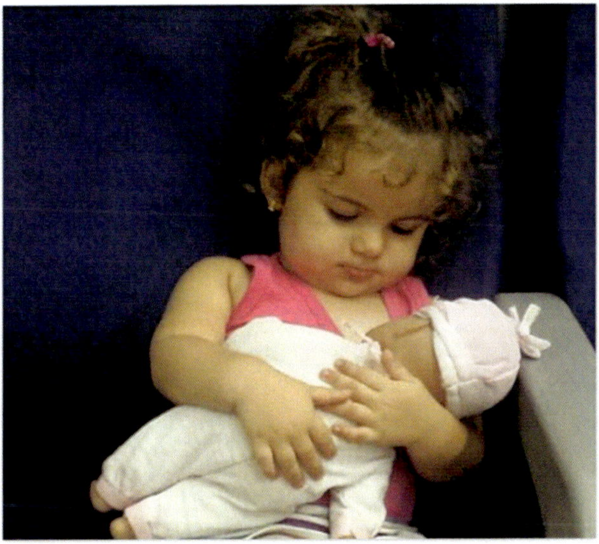

Photo 2-1: Playing at breastfeeding the baby
Source: Perrando Hospital. Resistencia, Chaco. Argentina.

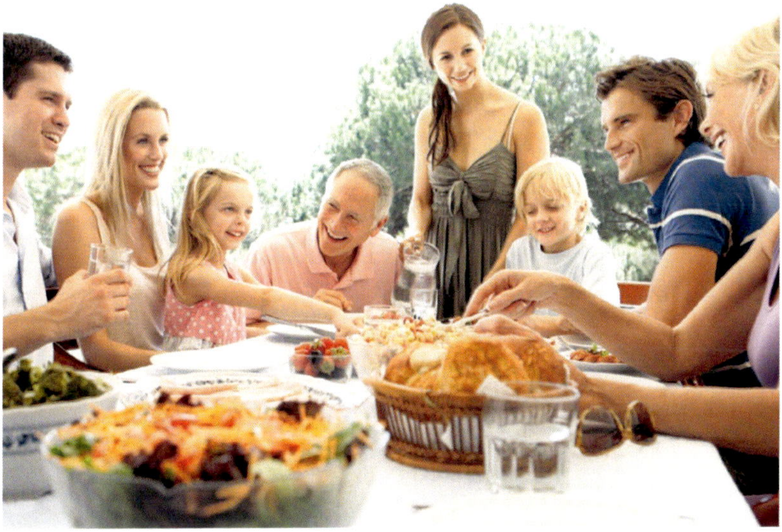

Photo 2-2: Food used for social integration

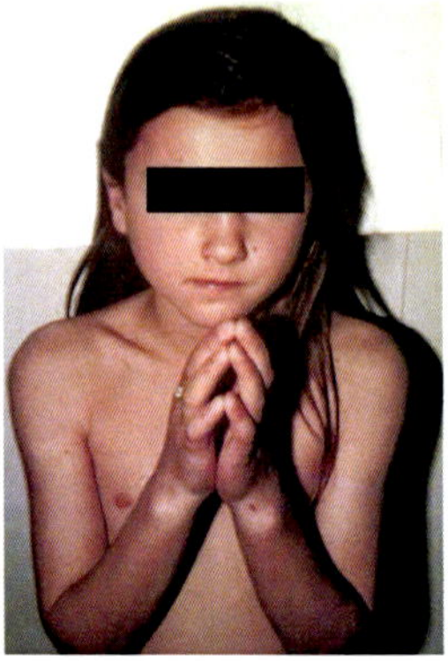

Joint mobility limitation

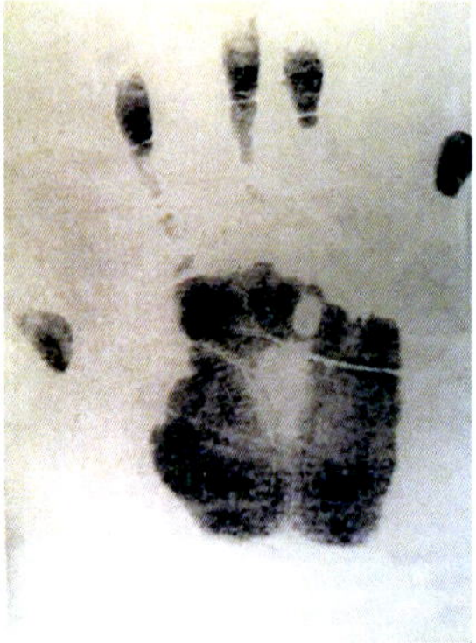

Lack of marking of the first phalanges

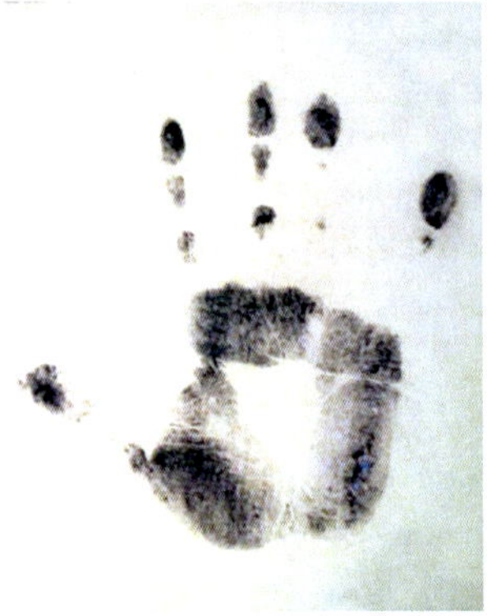

Diabetics without kidney disease

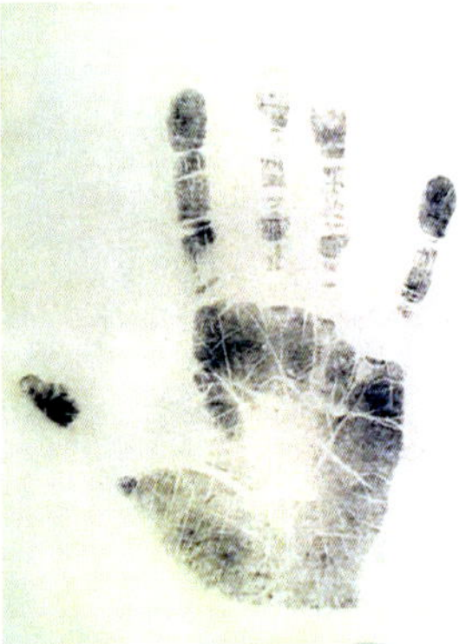

Normal control

Photo 4-1: Diabetic nephropathy patient

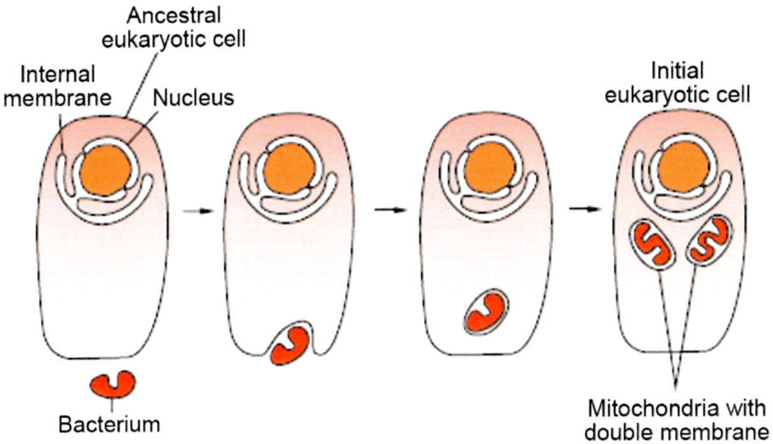

Fig. 4-1: Evolution from ancestral eukaryotic cells to mitochondrial integration

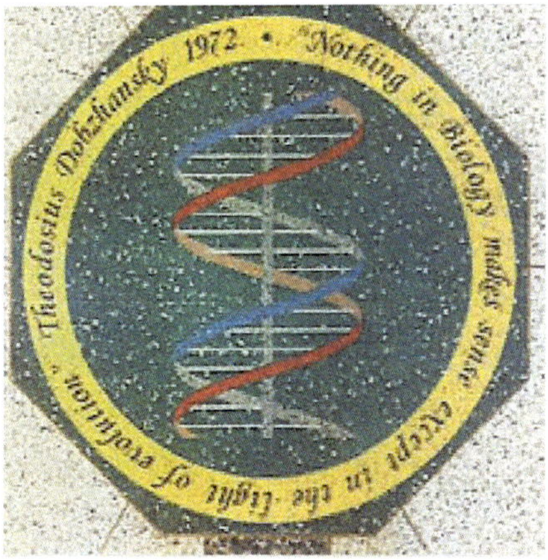

"Nothing in biology makes sense except in the light of evolution"
—Theodosius Dobzhansky

Photo 6-1: Medallion mosaic on the floor of the Jordan Hall of Science.
University of Notre Dame

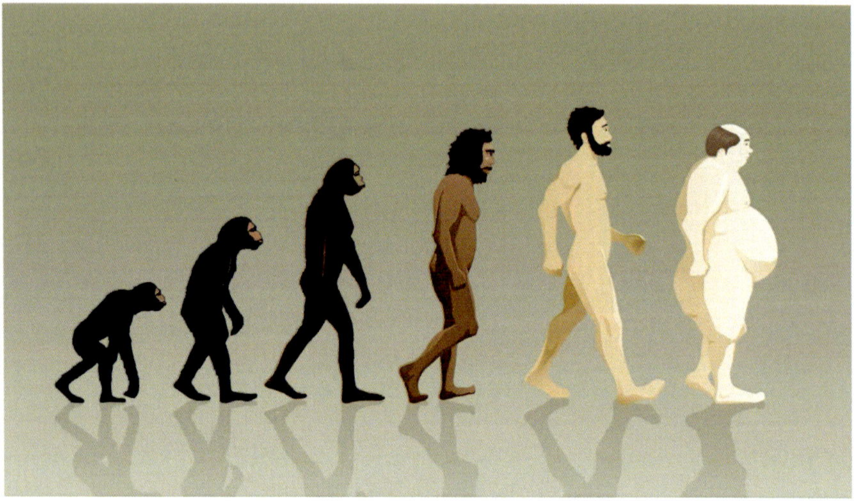

Fig. 6-1: Human evolution

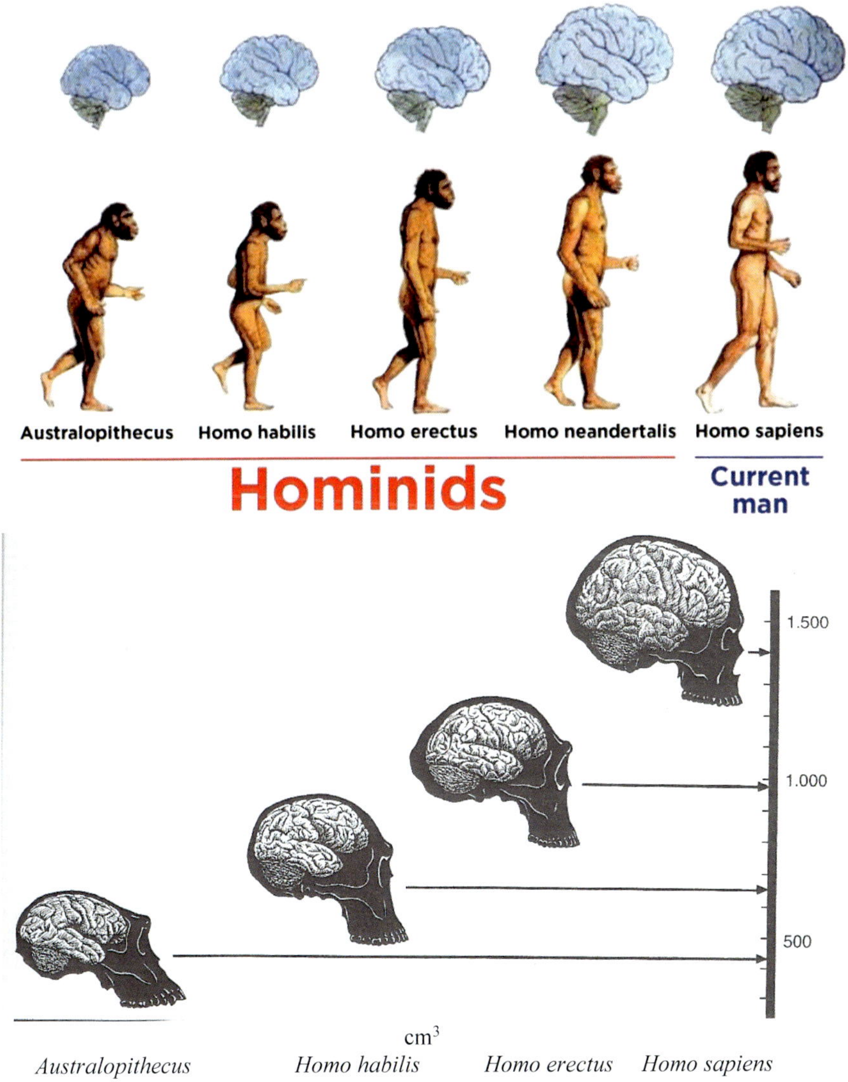

Fig. 6-2: Encephalization

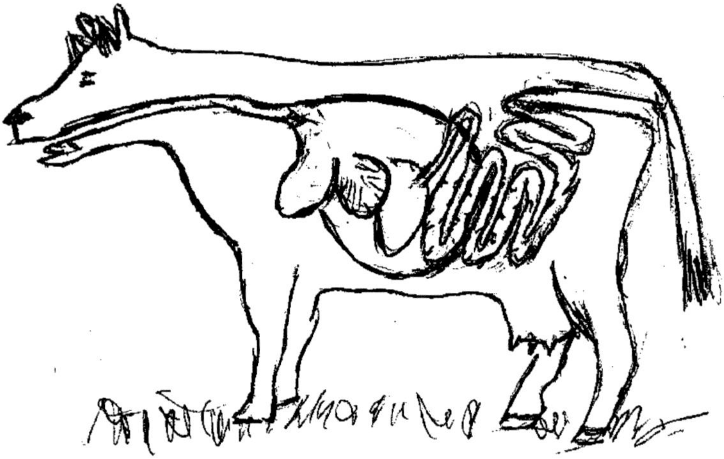

Fig. 6-3: Anatomy of the digestive system of the cow

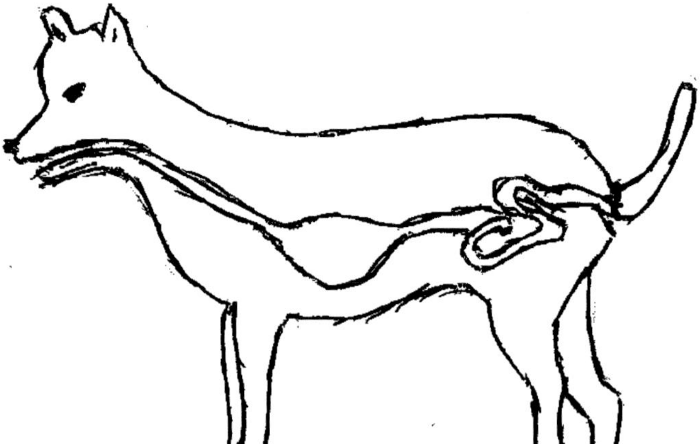

Fig. 6-4: Anatomy of the digestive system of the wolf

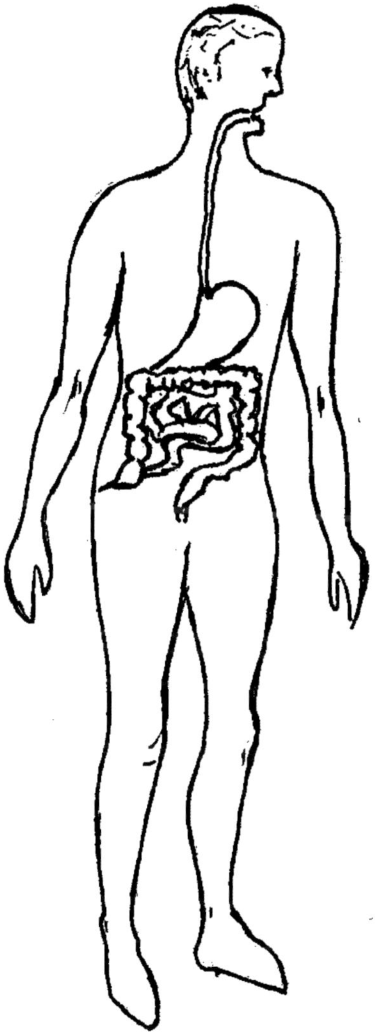

Fig. 6-5: Anatomy of the digestive system of a human.

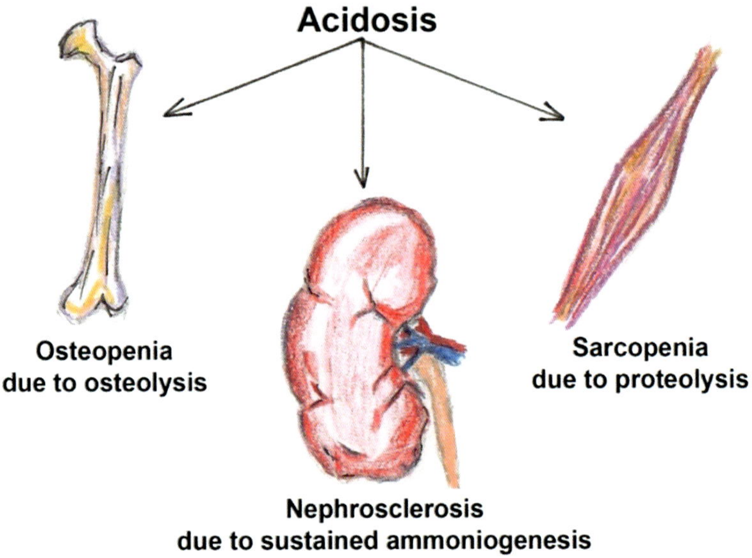

Fig. 7-1: Effect of acidosis on the skeletal, muscular and renal structure
Source: Voyer, Luis E. Medio interno. "Fisiología, patología y tratamiento de los líquidos orgánicos". Ed. Journal. Buenos Aires. 2017: 89 - 90.

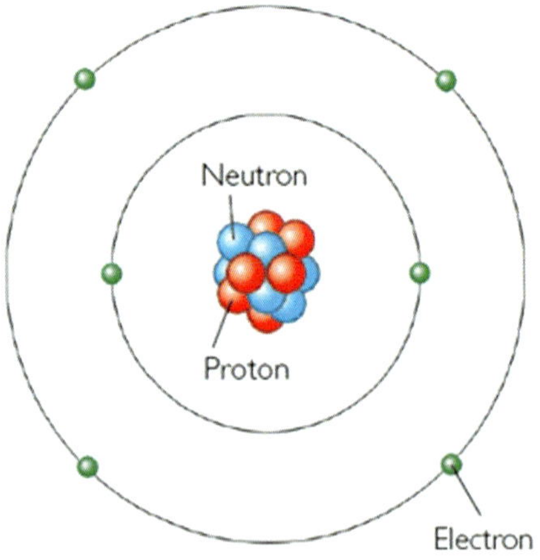

Protons: charges +. Electrons: charges

Fig. 7-2: Structure of an atom. Simplified bidimensional scheme

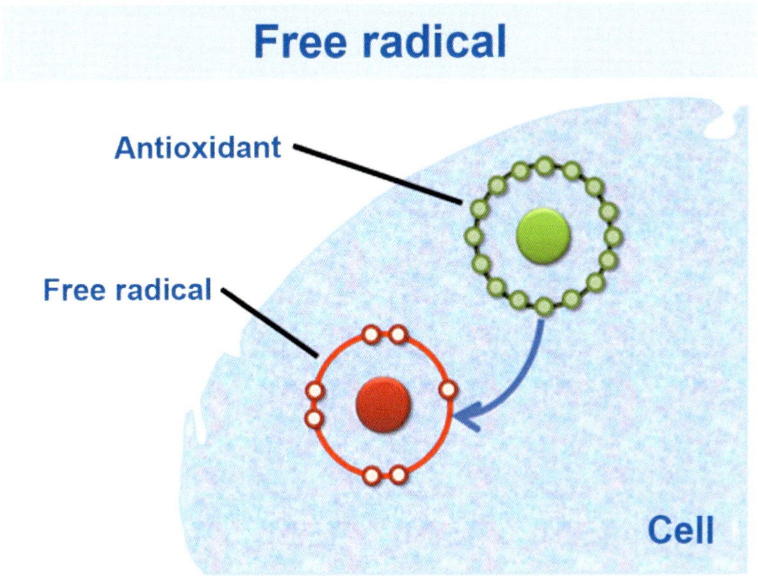

Fig. 7-3: Simplified bidimensional scheme

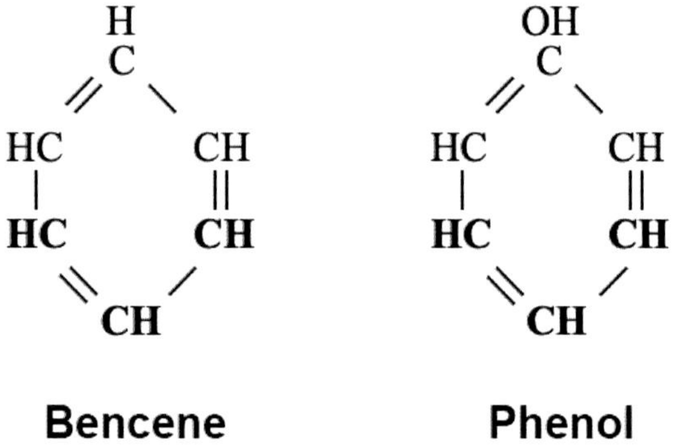
H
C
HC
CH
HC
CH
CH
Bencene
OH
C
HC
CH
HC
CH
CH
Phenol

Fig. 7-4

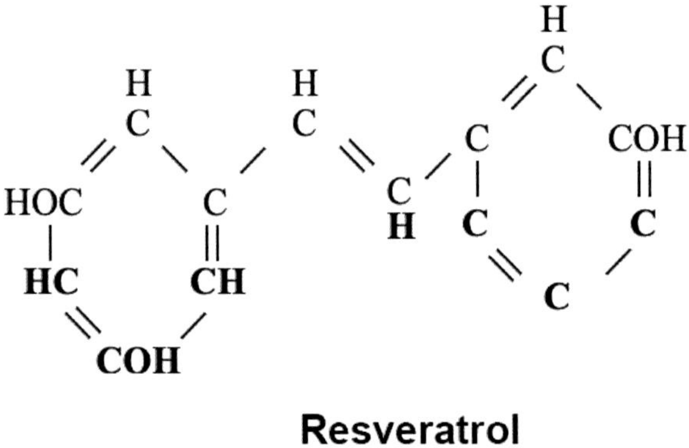
H
C
HOC
C
HC
CH
COH
H
C
C
H
H
C
C
COH
C
C
C
Resveratrol

Fig.7-5

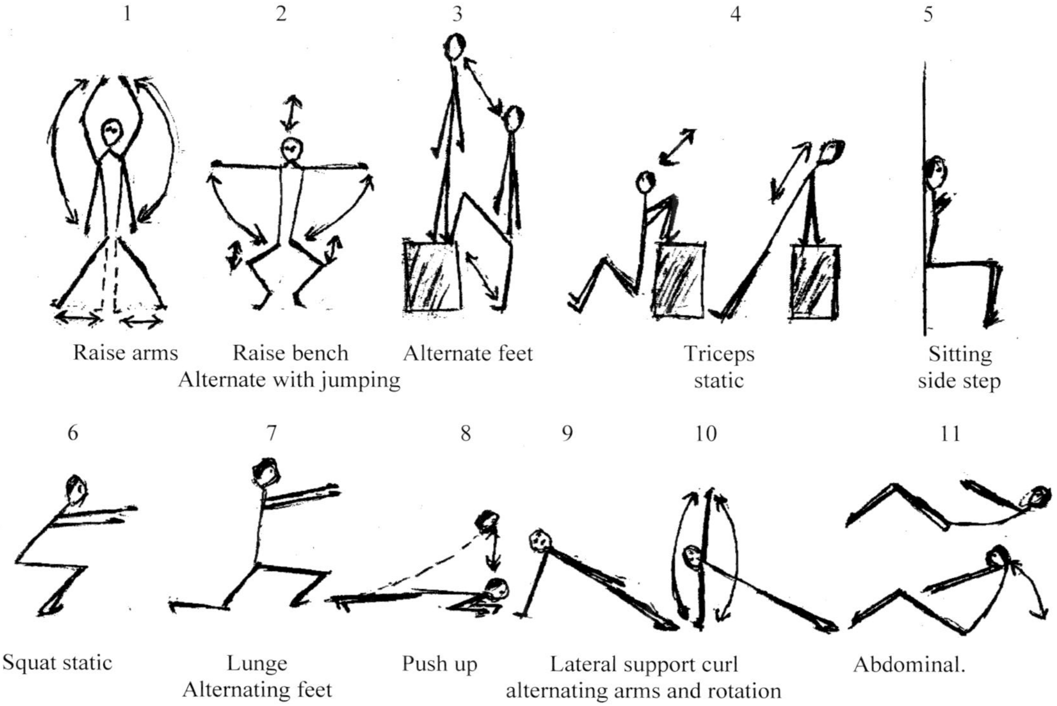
1
2
3
4
5
Raise arms
Raise bench
Alternate with jumping
Alternate feet
Triceps
static
Sitting
side step
6
7
8
9
10
11
Squat static
Lunge
Alternating feet
Push up
Lateral support curl
alternating arms and rotation
Abdominal.

12 13

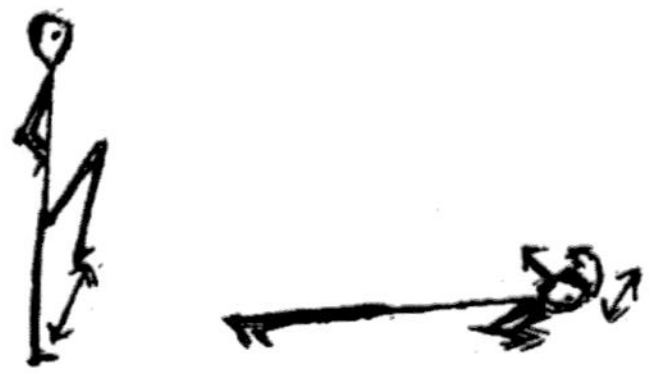

Alternating Static leaning on elbows and feet

Fig. 8-1: Gymnastics in 9 minutes
Based on the High-Intensity-Circuit-Training, H.I.C.T, by Chris Jordan

CHAPTER 1

MEALS FROM A NEW POINT OF VIEW

The role of food in the growth, development and repair of organs and tissues, and therefore in the preservation of health is already known, which in turn implies the prevention of diseases.

With the current knowledge of physiology, cellular structure and molecular biology, food today must be seen from a new dimension. It plays a fundamental role in the treatment of numerous diseases, adjunctive treatment not only with pharmacology, surgery and radiotherapy but also in the field of psychiatry, kinesiology, oncology and infectiology. All of this corrects underlying metabolic disorders that cause diseases, such as those derived from weight gain and obesity, allowing sustainable cures over time, avoiding recurrences or even from cancer and infections by correcting oxidative stress, chronic inflammation and modulating immunology. Apoptosis, the programmed cell death beginning at the development of the embryo, during life, allows the reuse of materials from aged cells and slows tumour development. Apoptosis partially depends on the intrinsic pathway of the mitochondria by increasing the permeability of their outer membrane, which releases cytochrome to the cytoplasm that activates apoptosis-activating proteins.

To maintain the functional integrity of the mitochondria so important for health, an alkaline diet is necessary. An acidic diet, which is most common, impairs mitochondrial function.

Currently, being overweight or obese, with its consequent diseases (mainly diabetes, hypertension and cardiovascular disease), is already an endemic and global problem in developed or developing countries, to which we must add cancer, osteoporosis and neurodegenerative diseases. This implies that a significant deterioration in the quality of life, a high social cost and the risk of a decrease in life expectancy is already evident. This has given rise to a certain boom in the so-called alternative 'medicines,' many outside the progress of science.

On the other hand, in 1989 in Japan, the concept of functional foods was proposed, a little elastic and somewhat debatable, which will be developed later.

It is important to implant the concept of the therapeutic power of food in the minds of the general population, to encourage it to see food from a new dimension as a means of treating diseases along with pharmacology, surgery and radiotherapy.

Ages of the human being, 1st, 2nd and 3rd

The **1st is childhood**, which paediatrics deals with.

Early childhood is defined as up to two years with breastfeeding as a priority, and second childhood is defined as over two years old, in which extra familial socialization with institutions begins.

Puberty and *a*dolescence are distinguished as being between 12 and 18 years of age. Adolescence is a critical period where the characteristics of childhood are lost and all the faculties of adults have not yet been acquired. Care must be taken with sexual development and consolidation or definition of gender. There is a greater vulnerability to accidents, drug addiction and social-work integration. With specialized assistance, adolescent medicine avoids risks and allows one to enter healthy adulthood where ethical development could be completed.

The **2nd is adulthood** dealt with by a doctor at a general medical practice.

The **3rd is old age** which geriatricians deal with. But the geriatrician especially faces age-related pathologies.

Just as adolescence is the final period of childhood with its own characteristics, of the transition to adulthood, there is a transition period from 60 years to the beginning of old age, which we could properly call *senescence.*

In this period of life, you may not have the capacity for any great exertions. There is a decrease in the body's ability to overcome very adverse situations and organic resilience, a greater vulnerability that must be compensated with prudence, a decrease in sexual potency and also less social integration due to, for example, retirement from work.

Specialized assistance in this period of life allows for the preservation of functions preventing cognitive deterioration in order to reach old age in good health and a state of bio-psycho-social well-being. Here it is essential to optimize nutrition, along with physical activity, mental work, normal sleep and preservation of a social openness that allows normal emotional exchanges.

Fermented foods are important in nutrition and even more than for younger age groups for microbiota and microbiome preservation. In addition, an alkaline diet is necessary to avoid subclinical acidosis with its consequent diseases, and bioactive phytochemicals that are beneficial to health, along with anti-oxidants, anti-inflammatory and anti-cancer compounds with preventive and co-adjuvant action in therapy for cardiovascular and neurodegenerative diseases, which are bio available through the adequate consumption of vegetables and fruit and the medicinal use of condiments.

An apple a day keeps the doctor away.

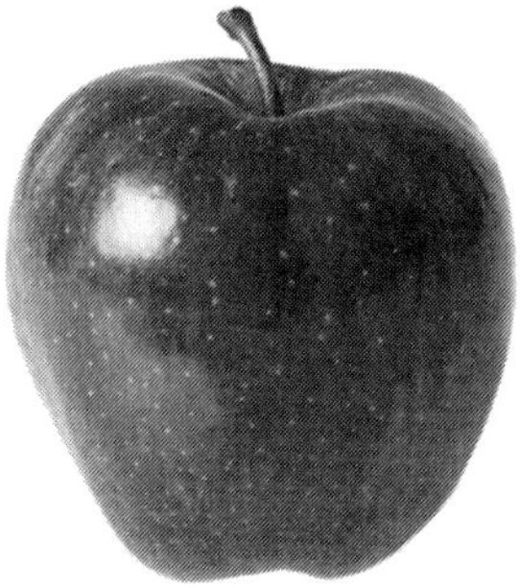

Photo 1-1: Apple

This anonymous saying does not refer precisely to the first apple Adam ate in Eden, the cause of so many later misfortunes! It is more that an apple, a symbol for all fruit and vegetables and natural foods that, together with meat and various spices, should be the basis of our usual diet; food that nature provides for us, and as far as possible, in its natural state.

A baked apple is no longer in its natural state, but its colour, aroma and flavour make it especially appetizing, and we can enjoy it occasionally but should never be a frequent part of our diet. Due to the high temperature during baking, it loses some of its vitamins and generates glycation products, also called glycotoxins, with undesirable health effects.

The aforementioned saying, to be more precise, should say: an apple a day *in its natural state*, keeps the doctor away. And the natural state is also like Adam ate it, without peeling it. In addition to the basic nutritional compounds, mainly glucides (misnamed carbohydrates) it contains chemical compounds with a small molecular weight called phytochemicals, which are typical of the plant kingdom, with important beneficial actions for health and flavonoids such as quercetin with anti-cancer and anti-allergic actions. These compounds are especially in the skin of the apple and are inactivated by heat.

In the anonymous saying above, "keeps the doctor away" is a fallacy because it considers the doctor as the one who only cures the disease, but the doctor must also prevent the disease. Health preservation and disease prevention should make the doctor a great health educator, seeking to change disease behaviours for health behaviours, among which is eating behaviour, and the way to achieve this is through education.

As far as food education is concerned, there is another saying, less well known:

"If man made it, don't eat it". But this should not be taken in an absolute sense. This saying is not anonymous but belongs to Jack LaLanne, a fitness expert and pioneer in health and an innovator in diet and nutrition.[1,2]

The content of this saying is in line with the previous one, about natural foods for normal meals without excluding foods from regional cuisines of different cultures for family or social events, such as a birthday cake, Christmas sweet bread, weekend ravioli or a pizza with friends, as part of an occasional meal but not as part of our everyday meals.

Among glucides are those not digested by gastrointestinal juices; fibres that in the intestine act as prebiotics favouring the development of intestinal bacterial flora.

Fibre fermentation bacteria produce saturated lipid acids, including butyric acid, which is not provided by food and is the main nutrient of enterocytes, the cells of the intestinal epithelium. In this way, a healthy intestine optimally fulfils its dual function: absorption of nutrients and acting as a barrier to toxins and pathogenic bacteria that cause disease.

This has resulted in a medical article, which paraphrases the aforementioned saying "*An apple a day, keeps the doctor away*", that was entitled: "An apple a day, keeps microbes away?" because a normal microbiota protects against microbes that can cause disease.

What should we eat? What is the healthiest *diet?*[3]

This is one of the topics that have been very relevant for several years; first because of the health risks of various diets for losing weight, some so absurd that they do not deserve consideration, and especially because of the awareness that for many chronic diseases such as diabetes, cardiovascular disease, neurodegenerative diseases and cancer, diet plays an important role in their prevention and control.

To end with paradigmatic axioms on food, we must remember the statement from the father of medicine (in Greco-Roman culture) Hippocrates, 400 years before Christ: *"Medicate yourself with food; do not feed yourself with medicines,"* a statement of special importance today.

Undoubtedly, numerous diseases require drugs, such as antibiotics for mainly bacterial or some viral infections, hormones for some glandular deficiencies such as insulin in type 1diabetes or corticosteroids for certain kidney diseases and highly inflammatory conditions. Abuse and self-medication, for example with antibiotics, antacids, digestives, analgesics, anxiolytics and other symptomatic medications are also undoubted. Medicating with food refers to the fact that a good diet prevents many diseases, as it improves defences by strengthening the immune system, favours digestion avoiding acidity and gastrointestinal disorders such as diarrhoea, constipation, intestinal polyps, decreases the risk of colorectal cancer and other organs and influences the emotional state. The intestine is well considered the second brain due to its extensive neural network interconnected with the central nervous system.

'Do not feed yourself with drugs' is also currently widely valid. Consumption of not just complementary drugs but also the aptly named nutritional supplements, poly-vitamins, minerals, synthetic fibre, protein powder such as bovine whey albumin, energizers and creatine, for muscle development.

Processed, and especially ultra-processed foods, also have multiple unnecessary additives for health, used for the conservation and greater acceptance in the market but have doubtful effects on health if they are part of our usual meals.

Consumption of ultra-processed foods such as sweets, biscuits, cakes and sweetened beverages, as a food base for adults over 60, increases the risk of chronic metabolic diseases, cancer and mortality.[4]

The overwhelming technology and industry developments achieved today make a careful evaluation necessary, within an ethical framework, of the advances that we must incorporate to achieve health and well-being in line with ecological environment preservation, but when in doubt, apply the precautionary principle; abstain and look for valid alternatives with more benefits and fewer risks.

There is a need for a greater intercommunication link between the food and the health industries, subordinating economic interests to an ethical framework for the good of our health.

Wendel Berry, an American writer, farmer and advocate of organic farming states: "People are fed by the food industry, which does not pay attention to health and they are treated by the health industry which does not pay attention to food."[5] It is universally recognized that food is a fundamental factor for health, preventing its deterioration. Consequently, food is an important factor that intervenes in longevity and even more importantly, in the quality of our lives.

With the current knowledge of physiology, cell structure, molecular biology, genetics and epigenetics, we can avoid situations that cause numerous diseases due to cellular damage that we now refer to, which will be dealt with extensor in respective chapters.

Situations that cause numerous diseases

Oxidative stress

Inflammatory chronicity

Mild and persistent acid-base imbalance

Depletion of mitochondrial metabolism by xenobiotics and acidosis

Oxidative stress

For growth, repair and specific organic functions, the energy for chemical reactions that make up the metabolism is of vital importance.

The availability of energy comes from oxidation><reduction, a metabolic process called redox, between atoms of reactive substances. Oxidation means the loss of one or more electrons, which generates so-called free radicals. Free radicals, oxidized atoms, are very reactive, seeking in fractions of a second to recover the lost electrons, which is called reduction. These electrons, not being free, are taken from other atoms, which in turn oxidize.

Oxidized atoms acted as *oxidants*.

The greatest production of energy in our cells is carried out in the mitochondria, where there are electron transport chains, the energy being stored in adenosine triphosphate (ATP) molecules.

In cells, there are *antioxidant* substances, the main one being glutathione, which gives up electrons preventing oxidation in other substances. *Glutathione* can reduce itself using the enzyme glutathione reductase.

The predominance of oxidation over reduction, surpassing the capacity of cellular antioxidants such as glutathione and other compounds, if it is mild, is good for the immune system and to kill pathogens, but if it is intense, it configures *oxidative stress*. Oxidative stress is an important factor in cellular damage participating in the pathogenesis of more than 100 diseases such as atherosclerosis, neurodegenerative diseases (Parkinson's, Alzheimer`s, Huntington's), metabolic diseases and even ageing and cell death. Situations such as infectious diseases, cancer, smoking or extreme physical exercise favour oxidative stress. Oxidative stress causes organic damage; it can be compared to oxidative damage in metals that undergo corrosion. To avoid oxidative stress, have a measured life with healthy behaviours and habits and among these, the regular intake of exogenous antioxidants, mainly flavonoid and non-flavonoid polyphenols and other phytochemicals abundant in fruit, vegetables and infusions with natural products are very beneficial for health.

Inflammatory chronicity

Inflammation is a defensive, normal and controlled reaction of the body to harmful agents—physical such as trauma, chemicals such as acids or biological such as infections by bacteria, viruses, fungi or parasites, subject to intensity, time and place. Problems arise when the inflammatory process is in a generalized and permanent state, causing or aggravating numerous diseases, such as obesity, diabetes, cardiovascular disease, arthritis and even cancer, which require adjuvant anti-inflammatory medication. Modulation of the potential capacity of an inflammatory process depends to a great extent on the diet, mainly as regards the quality of the lipids, since there are pro-inflammatory and anti-inflammatory ones. The constituent acids of lipids, generally called *fatty acids*, are preferably referred to as *lipid acids.* Lipid acids are from sea or land animal and vegetable origin and are pro-inflammatory or anti-inflammatory, with variable bioavailability according to absorption and metabolization, and they are more or less stable according to susceptibility to oxidation, depending on the presence or not of antioxidants. A balance is necessary, as it is risky to almost nullify the capacity for inflammatory reaction, an excessive and persistent inflammatory state is the conditioning and aggravating factor in many diseases. Choosing the best quality lipids that we incorporate into our usual diet to optimize it will have invaluable benefits for health.

Mild and persistent acid-base imbalance

The acid-base state of our internal environment, considered as the organic liquids that surround our cells, is alkaline, with a pH of 7.4 with very narrow variations, between 7.35 and 7.45. These values are maintained by the buffering effect of bicarbonate, the alkaline reserves of the bones, the capacity for acid elimination in the urine and the respiratory elimination of carbon dioxide. In this aspect of the regulation of the internal environment, maintaining normal values of pH, bicarbonate and carbon dioxide, food is also of paramount importance, which is often not taken into account and consequently generally neglected, with far-reaching consequences over the years. According to the quality of our food, we distinguish a diet being acidic or alkaline by the number of acid residues that these foods leave when metabolized. In the industrialized countries of the Western world, 50% of the acid load of the organism comes from the food, however, normal values of pH, bicarbonate and carbon dioxide are maintained at the expense of a permanent consumption of plasma bicarbonate which is replaced by calcium carbonate from the bones, but calcium is lost by the kidney. Together with this, there is a permanent state of urinary acidification and ammonia production by the kidney to eliminate hydrogen ions using glutamine from the muscle mass. This leads over the years to an increased risk of bone demineralization, loss of muscle mass and kidney failure.

To improve our diet with an important intake of alkaline foods, reducing at the same time the acid contributions, means to preserve the state of health over the years as explained in the respective topics (Chapter 7).

The depletion of mitochondrial metabolism by xenobiotics

With the great development of industries, mainly chemical and pharmaceutical, the environmental pollution of air, land and sea and the availability of cosmetic and medicinal products create a great potential for exposure to non-biological products, that is *xenobiotics*, such as mercury, bisphenols, phthalates, dioxins, herbicides, pesticides, synthetic sweeteners (some of which have petroleum derivatives), analgesics, anxiolytics and synthetic antibiotics, which can interfere with vital structures and functions and especially to the microbiota and structure and function of mitochondria.

Reducing the consumption of ultra-processed foods to a minimum, avoiding the abuse of antibiotics and self-medication preserves a normal metabolism, thus avoiding serious diseases. On the other hand, optimal meals, together with a healthy lifestyle, are the basis for changing a disease behaviour into a health behaviour through which, in addition, gene transcription is modulated by epigenetic factors and improves the immune status.

Health and disease behaviours

With reference to health and disease behaviours, they are shown on the graph with a fork, feet and fingers.

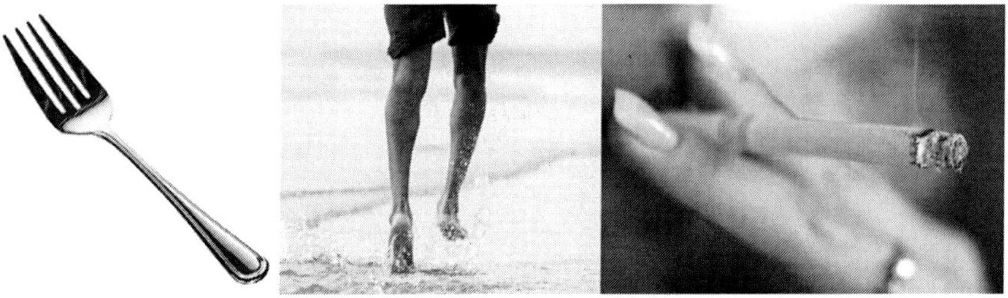

Photo 1-2: Factors that make up health or disease behaviours

The fork refers to food, the feet are a symbol of activity and the fingers as a symbol of habits, referring to one of the most harmful, the habit of smoking. To this must be added the environment, or the ecosystem where we live, which must be preserved. Changing some habits is difficult. Since it is difficult to quit smoking, is also difficult to change your diet. We eat according to whether 'I like it' or 'I don't like it'. But you are not born with tastes, they are acquired, the only taste you are born knowing is breast milk. Educate your body. The body listens: thoughts are the seeds of action, be aware of what you say to yourself.

The body listens and believes what you say, so take care of what you say, eliminate self-sabotage, don't say "I can't"; say "I want it", "I can't do it, but I'm going to achieve it". Defend your goals, and write them down, with a figure in your mind.

All hypnosis is self-hypnosis.

The body listens.

Microbiota and microbiome

We live with the microbiota, a set of microorganisms, mainly bacteria (70%) and fungi, mostly from our intestinal flora, in a number 10 times greater than the number of our cells, which is 30 billion. Microbiota is largely derived from food that germinates on the ground, but begins at the moment of natural birth, (not by caesarean) and continues with intimate contact through breast milk.

Herbicides and pesticides, which do not attack crops, (and even less, transgenic crops), sterilize the soils affect the nutritional value of food and compromise our microbiota.

The fibre in food is one of the main factors that favour the development of the microbiota, therefore called prebiotics, to which are added microorganisms by fermented foods, thereafter called probiotics.

Metabolic products and genes, which are nucleic acids from the microbiota and food, constitute the microbiome, which interacts with the genes of our genome.

Mitochondria

We are the evolutionary result of interactions with the environment. Mitochondria, the largest organelles in our cells (Fig. 1-1) are the metabolic centres for 90 to 95% of energy production. According to a solid evolutionary theory, mitochondria are aerobic bacteria, that is, with an oxygen-dependent metabolism incorporated into the cell structure approximately one billion years ago. Our state of health depends largely on the balance in this symbiotic coexistence, and its imbalance implies an important role in the origin and mechanism, etiopathogeneses of numerous diseases, such as cardiovascular, neurological, neurodegenerative, metabolic, early ageing, cancer and others.[6,7]

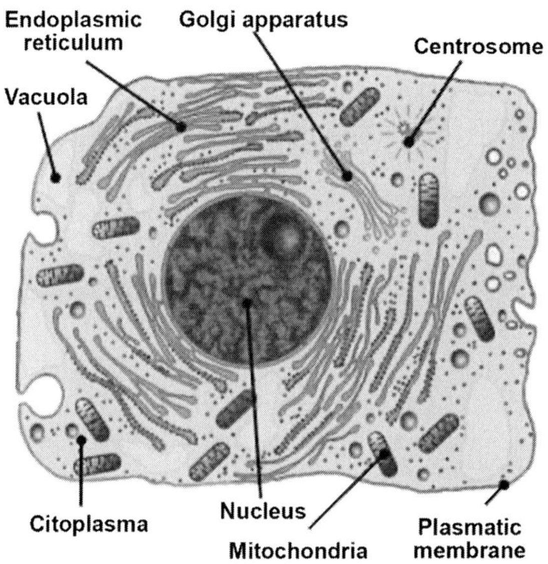

Fig. 1-1: A cell with the nucleus and organelles

Mitochondria, like the bacteria of the microbiota, have a prokaryotic cell structure, do not have a nucleus and nucleic acids are in the cytoplasm, and their metabolism is aerobic. Both are exposed to damage in their integrity and function due to the action of non-biological compounds, therefore called xenobiotics, such as antibiotics, analgesics, or non-steroid anti-inflammatory drugs (NSAIDs).

Genetics

Our genetic inheritance is encoded mainly in the DNA of the nucleus of the cell, the nuclear DNA, of paternal and maternal transmission through the sperm and the ovule, but there is also DNA in the mitochondria from an exclusively maternal transmission. Mitochondrial DNA is transmitted exclusively by the mother, since in fertilization only the head of the sperm with the nuclear DNA enters the maternal cell, leaving the tail and neck of the sperm, where the mitochondria are, outside the egg.

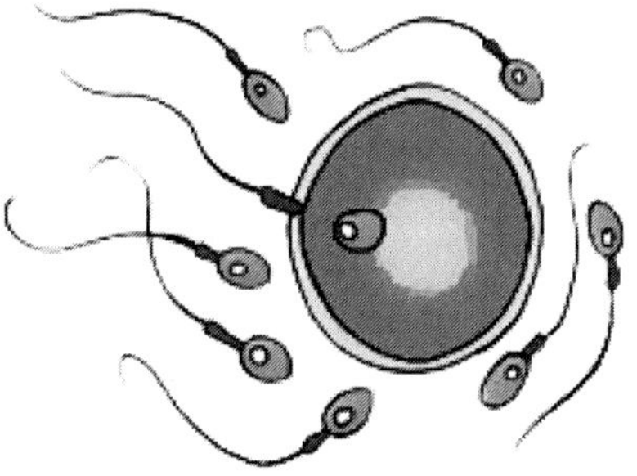

Fig. 1-2: Fecundation

Mitochondrial DNA represents only 0.1% of the total genetic material in our cells, but alterations in this genetic material constitute a causal or leading factor, by various mechanisms, of various diseases.

Unlike nuclear DNA, which is only 90% genetically encoded, all mitochondrial DNA is genetically encoded. In addition, nuclear DNA is provided with histones and proteins that in addition to intervening in gene expression have a structural packaging protection function against eventual damage. Mitochondrial DNA does not have histones and is, therefore, more easily exposed to damage by various factors in addition to xenobiotics, for instance, damage from oxidative stress. From DNA, genetic codes are transmitted by transcripts into the RNA messenger throughout the cell for expression in protein synthesis. A large part of our genome is not coding, and its function was unknown; today we know that to a large extent they activate or deactivate genetic codes in interaction with components of the microbiome.

Epigenetics

Activating or inhibiting factors for expression and development act on the vast majority of the conditions of genetic inheritance. All these factors that act over genetics constitute what is called epigenetics. Epigenetic factors come from the microbiome and the ecological and socio-cultural environment. Even though that has not yet been understood in all its significance, it deserves to be highlighted that the tremendous complexity of neural networks of our brain means that emotions and thoughts, without yet fully understanding their mechanisms, can also act as epigenetic factors beyond the conditioning of habits and behaviours. It is interesting to analyze what happens with the overweight and the obese and the consequent metabolic syndrome, where there are families in which parents and children suffer from it. Genetic conditioning may exist, but for no more than 10% and it manifests itself only with an eating behaviour that favours it, as it exists at high risk in an obesogenic environment.

In other pathologies such as hypercholesterolemia, arterial hypertension, cardiovascular disease, breast or prostate cancer, a hereditary predisposition due to genetic conditioning may also exist, but it is not an obligatory determinant if there are no triggering factors, such as lifestyle and cultural habits, and, of utmost importance, food.

We are in the post-genomic era after the achievements of the human genome project. Today we know that we have around 25,000 genes, instead of the presumed 100,000, to encode approximately 200,000 proteins (proteome). The idea of 1 gene, 1 protein and 1 cellular behaviour is no longer valid. A gene has pleiotropic expression and it can be expressed in numerous proteins. Proteins, after their gene translation, are modified by union with other molecules such as sugars, and by glycosylation; also with lipids, phosphate or acids, which modifies their biological activity by modulating their function.

The microbiota and the microbiome, which act very early, as environmental and cultural factors that can act on stability and gene translation, constitute epigenetics factors.[8,9]

Genes are not the only ones responsible for what happens to us, but everything that acts over them, and we are partly responsible for the factors to which we expose our genes. Most of our normal or pathological characteristics are of multifactorial origin, that is, polygenic. Polygenic is understood as not many genes but many determining factors, genetics and epigenetics. Among epigenetics factors, the relevance of nutrition has led to what is called nutrigenomics.

Social inheritance

> "It is not true that all inheritance is measured by nuclear DNA. A well-documented example is cultural evolution."[10]

In addition to the genetic inheritance encoded in DNA, we have social inheritance, that is, culture, encoded in society and that reaches each child in the first place through the family, which is like the RNA messenger in genetic inheritance. Eating behaviour is part of social inheritance, and education acts on that basis. The mother has a special intervention not only in genetic inheritance, in which she contributes in addition to nuclear DNA with mitochondrial DNA but also in social inheritance due to the special relationship with the child in the first two years of life, mainly due to the intimate implicit contact from the practice of breastfeeding.[11,12]

CHAPTER 2

EATING BEHAVIOURS

Breastfeeding

The period of *breastfeeding* is of fundamental importance for the health of the child and the entire future of its growth and development, with repercussions even into adult life. The insurmountable benefits of breastfeeding lie not only in the quality of the milk specific to the species but also in other factors that are still only partially known today.[13,14]

With breastfeeding, there are benefits for the growth and development of the child due to factors beyond the purely organic ones, due to the close mother-child bond that it creates, with repercussions not yet fully understood of its transcendent significance.

There is a culture of breastfeeding for which paediatricians, childcare providers, pediatric hospitals, and general hospitals (recognized as 'baby-friendly hospitals'), which national and international medical societies such as the WHO and UNICEF are working towards. For more than 40 years there have been attempts to eradicate the culture of artificial lactation that we still occasionally see, with girls play-acting with their dolls like a mother giving a baby a bottle.

It is striking that just as you see children playing the role of doctors and patients, you do not see girls imitate their mothers by putting a doll on their chests.

Could it be that somehow a message of misplaced modesty is transmitted to them about it?

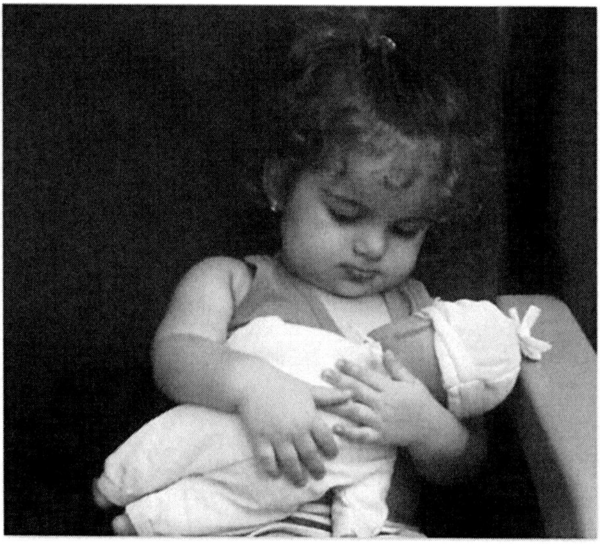

Photo 2-1: Playing at breastfeeding the baby
Source: Perrando Hospital. Resistencia, Chaco. Argentina.

Optimal nutrition should begin with breastfeeding and be supplemented from the sixth month with the gradual introduction of various nutrients until reaching a varied adult diet. In many industrialized countries only 60% of infants receive exclusive breastfeeding up to two months of age, and between 30 and 40% up to 6 months. The WHO has set a goal of reaching 50% by 2025. After six months, together with complementary meals, efforts should be made to maintain breastfeeding for up to two years of age. Breastfeeding does not need to be replaced by substitutes in no more than 4% of cases. In the few cases of contraindication to breastfeeding, the provision of human milk from banks should be sought first.

Human milk banks

The WHO accredited human milk banks as one of the best health strategies for reducing infant mortality and protecting breastfeeding. The Human Milk Banking Association of North America, the European Milk Bank Association and the Ibero-American Network of Human Milk Banks have been organized. These centres work with selected donor mothers with various collection points. The milk is analysed, pasteurized and frozen and used especially for premature children and those with high-risk diseases. The implementation of breastfeeding with human milk in these children has shown evident benefits with a decrease in the incidence of sepsis and between 58 and 77% of necrotizing enteritis in preterm infants and consequently, a decrease in mortality. With breastfeeding, in addition to the benefits referred to in premature infants, there are fewer sudden deaths, allergies, asthma and atopic dermatitis and 52% less coeliac disease, when the introduction of gluten is carried out while the child is still breastfeeding.

Likewise, in children who received at least three months of exclusive breastfeeding, a 30% decrease in type 1 diabetes and a 40% decrease in type 2 diabetes was observed, related to between 15 and 30% less obesity. With six months or more of exclusive breastfeeding, 20% less acute lymphocytic leukaemia and 15% less acute myeloid leukaemia were also observed.

Breastfeeding supplies the child with living tissue that has antibodies, mainly surface antibodies, in immunoglobulin (Ig) A (IgA) together with macrophages, lysozyme and lactoferrin, all of them with antimicrobial actions. Breastfeeding also means benefits for the health of the mother, among others, a lower risk of premenopausal breast cancer.[15]

Breastfed children show a lower incidence of otitis and diarrhoea. Breastfeeding has always been and continues to be the optimal meal for infants since breast milk is the ideal food to promote growth and development, not only due to its protein/caloric intake but also due to its hormonal content such as insulin, estrogens, androgens and growth factors. Breastfeeding promotes the maturing process of the intestinal wall. The lactation period was extended in ancient times to around three years, supplemented with solid and semi-solid foods. Faced with the occasional early maternal death, some children were fed by other mothers.

When provision from breast milk banks is not feasible, substitutes will only be used, such as modified cow's milk, or almond milk, of which there are very good quality varieties manufactured by the food industry. It can also be prepared at home as described in Chapter 9. Human milk substitutes are never better or even the same and should be considered medicinal foods subject to medical prescription. After the lactation period, milk and its derivatives are not essential foods, which will be considered extensively later.

Among the achievements of the medical societies that addressed the problem, the most outstanding was the campaign of the pediatric societies, within the framework of the WHO and UNICEF, and the United Nations who challenged companies that produce breast milk substitutes, liquid or powdered modified cow's milk, or any other infant food supplied with a bottle or that was indicated to replace all or part of breast milk.

With this challenge and with the objective of protecting and promoting breastfeeding, the International Code of Marketing of Breastmilk Substitutes was signed.[16] It was approved by the World Health Assembly in 1981 and ratified in 1996. The WHO also determined the denomination as "medicine" for infant formulas and therefore their employment must be supported by medical reasons. We refer below to some of its most relevant content.

It sets standards for marketing, sales, advertising, the spaces in which they are displayed and relationships with health agents and their associations.

It does not allow any publicity intended for the public, nor donation of samples or contributions to mothers, relatives, health agents or medical institutions.

Product labels must clearly state that breastfeeding is superior.

Breast milk substitute products, such as food and medicine, should only be provided as indicated by health agents.[17]

Beyond the period of breastfeeding, and with the importance of the things that are promoted from childhood, to establish life habits and eating behaviour for a lifetime, the consumption of natural foods that provide proteins, fibre, vitamins and minerals should be encouraged. Processed foods and sugary beverages that are of low nutritional value, poor in fibre and with excessive calories, salt and sugar or fructose syrup should be limited.

Composition of human milk

In the composition of human milk, 60% of the protein is made up of whey protein, and lactalbumin (albuminous milk). Regarding lipids, between 53 and 58% of the lipid acids are polyunsaturated with a high content, 346mg%, of essential lipid acids, linoleic and alpha-linolenic.

It is worth highlighting the presence of long-chain omega-6 arachidonic acid (AA) and omega-3 *docosahexaenoic acid* (DHA) with a low omega-6/omega-3 index. The DHA present in mother's milk (and which is absent in cow's milk or other animals) is important for brain cell growth, postnatal myelination and cognitive and visual development. DHA does not burn like lipid; it is structural to cells and makes up 50% of the fat in the brain. It should be remembered that brain development is very intense especially in the last trimester of pregnancy and during the first two years of life. The mother provides these long-chain lipid acids with a low omega- 6/omega-3 index through the placenta during pregnancy and later through breastfeeding, and consumption of fish must be introduced because of its high content of DHA. Omega-3 and omega-6 lipid acids are polyunsaturated and are unstabilised by the effects of light and heat. The hepatic biosynthesis capacity, although it is also present in the foetus and newborn baby, due to functional immaturity is insufficient for this stage of great growth and development. These acids have a direct action on the integrity of the nervous system, DHA and AA are present in the membranes of brain cells and their concentration strongly increases during the development of the central nervous system in the last trimester of gestation and during the first year of life.[18]

With reference to glucides, (misnamed carbohydrates), beta-lactose predominates in human milk, which conditions the development of the intestinal bacterial flora with the Bifidus bacillus, the Bifidobacterium longum that protects the infant from pathogenic bacteria such as Escherichia coli. Besides this, there are antibodies, mainly surface antibodies, in IgA, together with macrophages, lysozyme and lactoferrin, all of them with antimicrobial action.

Calcium and magnesium and the trace elements iron, copper and zinc have a high bioavailability in human milk. The calcium/phosphorus ratio of 2:1 favours the absorption of calcium. Iron absorption from human milk is high at 49%. The low sodium and chlorine content is adequate for the lower urinary concentrating capacity of the infant. To all this, it must be added that breastfeeding promotes the maturing process of the intestinal wall.

Cow's milk and dairy products

The total or partial replacement of the mother's milk in an infant's meals with cow's milk means the contribution of a heterologous protein, consisting of 80% casein (casein milk) and 20% whey protein, which determines an immunological reaction that produces an inflammatory state of the intestinal mucosa that can lead to loss of occult blood in faecal matter and a delay in the maturing of the intestinal epithelium.

Seventy per cent of lipids are saturated mainly palmitic acid. The essential lipid acid content is only 99mg%, significantly less than the 346mg% of human milk.

Long-chain polyunsaturated AA and DHA, which have already been mentioned for their importance for the growth of brain cells and postnatal myelination, are absent from cow's milk.

With regard to minerals, there is a higher proportion of phosphorus than calcium, which decreases the absorption of calcium, and the bioavailability of magnesium and the trace elements iron, copper and zinc is also lower. Iron absorption from cow's milk is only 10%, significantly less than 49% in the case of human milk. Chloride and sodium content is high for the infant's urinary concentrating capacity.

Loss of occult blood in stools produced by the inflammatory state of the intestinal mucosa, induced by the immunological reaction to the heterologous protein, i.e. the casein from cow's milk, is the cause of iron deficiency anaemia in infants, which has led in recent years to the dairy industry adding iron to milk, which may compensate for losses induced by it.

The consumption of cow's milk, in addition to producing an allergy to it, probably in genetically predisposed subjects, is a triggering factor of autoimmune mechanisms by generating antibodies not only against casein but also against insulin and insulin growth factor. These antibodies can attack organs such as the intestine, thyroid and pancreas.[19-21] Many works investigate this aspect and the relationship that may exist between childhood diabetes and other pathologies.

The most widely accepted hypothesis is that because breastfeeding promotes the maturing of the intestinal wall, the absence or limitation of it hinders intestinal maturing, which would explain not only the manifest allergy to cow's milk in some cases but also the powerful diabetogenicity observed in proteins of vegetable origin such as soya and wheat. Paradoxically, although cow's milk has a low glycemic index, the insulin response is high, favouring the incidences of insulin resistance.[22, 23]

The absence of long-chain omega-6 and omega-3 AA and DHA in cow's milk hinders the cognitive and visual development of the infant. Likewise, the high content of saturated lipid in cow's milk is possibly a conditioning factor for the increases in cholesterol and atherosclerosis lesions that can be observed early on in childhood. In this regard, researchers linked to the dairy industry seek to modify the fat content of cow's milk by changing the animals' feed.

The specificity of milk is given in the protein quality, which can lead to allergic reactions to the milk of another species and in the quality of the fats.

Cow's milk intolerance

In a large number of people, after the lactation period milk is not tolerated due to the inability to digest it because of the loss of intestinal lactase. Fermentation in the intestine of unabsorbed lactose determines abdominal distention, acidosis, diarrhoea with acidic stools and the risk of dehydration and malnutrition. The frequency of this disorder varies in different countries or ethnic groups, affecting 95% of white Americans, between 63% and 66% of African Americans, 52% of Americans of Mexican origin, 15% of Spaniards and only 1 or 3% of the Swedish and Danish. The decrease or loss of intestinal lactase after two or three years of age is a natural process since milk is the specific food for the period of lactation. The persistence of lactase activity throughout adult life, especially in Swedes and Danes, seems to be the result of a genetic change, a mutation that acts as an adaptive trait.[24]

Intolerance to cow's milk is caused by an allergic reaction to one of the 40 different proteins it contains. The most frequently sensitizing proteins that act as allergens are casein, alpha and beta lactalbumin, immunoglobulins, serum albumin, lactoperoxidase, alkaline phosphatase, and peroxidase and others and several of them can even act simultaneously. It is the most common food allergy in infants and children, affecting up to 7.5% of the child population and 4% of children under four years of age, and represents 25% of food allergies in childhood. The clinical manifestations can be cutaneous, respiratory or digestive and as varied as rashes, asthma, colitis, eosinophilic esophagitis, angioedema and severe anaphylaxis. The manifestations occur with the ingestion of milk, dairy products, foods that contain milk or protein hydrolysates or caseinates, even during breastfeeding when the mother ingests cow's milk. They tend to fade with age, but the forms mediated by immunoglobulin E can persist until adolescence and are rare in adulthood[25,26.] Epidemiological data also link the consumption of milk, not cheese or yoghurt, with acne in adolescents and young adults.[27-29]

The Nutrition Committee of the American Academy of Pediatrics, responding to the growing concern of many paediatricians about the potential risks of cow's milk as part of the habitual diet of children, created a communication entitled "Should Milk Drinking by Children Be Discouraged?" Also, in relation to this issue in paediatrics in 2002 is the article "Milk: Can a 'Good' Food Be So Bad?" Responding to this argument there are some arguments in favour and others against, with 46 bibliographic citations.[30] The point is that together with the indisputable recognition that no substitute is equal to breastfeeding, after the breastfeeding period that can extend beyond the second year, milk was considered for a long time as a priority food, especially for the growth of the child, but has now lost its role of dogma in health.

Something similar also happens in relation to the consumption of dairy products for the prevention of osteoporosis, especially in women. Cheeses and yoghurt, products of the artificial fermentation of milk, when metabolized leave strongly acidic residues, especially cheeses neutralized first by plasma bicarbonate and then by the strong alkaline reserves of bone, calcium carbonate. From the carbonate, the bicarbonate of the plasma is replaced and the calcium is lost through the urine. Today many producers add calcium to yoghurt.

Africans and African Americans consume less dairy and less calcium and suffer from less osteoporosis than the white population with its much higher intake of dairy, and consequently, calcium. It can be strongly questioned that dairy products, due to their calcium content, are a means of preventing osteoporosis.[31] Cheese and yoghurts are foods resulting from an artificial fermentation process with lactic acidification by bacteria and by enzymatic action. In this process, lactose is largely transformed, originating with lactic acid as the main product and acetaldehyde and diacetyl as a secondary product, leaving galactose remnants. This determines that cheeses and yoghurts are tolerated to a great extent in subjects who can no longer digest lactose.

Milk and dairy products can be contaminated like many other foods with dioxins, as a result of the use of herbicides and pesticides, or due to the proximity of industrial centres or urban waste incineration plants. Also, cardboard or plastic containers are a source of contamination.

Given that the dietary contributions of milk and dairy derivatives, fundamentally proteins and calcium, can be widely covered by meat, vegetables and fruit, milk and dairy derivatives should not be part of our usual diet, not even once a day.

Almond milk, already referred to when treating breastfeeding substitutes, is a recommended alternative to use in tea for breakfast and snacks, along with a vegetable and fruit salad. Eventually, you can use a little milk to make a white sauce with broccoli or cauliflower or eat a portion of cheese once or twice a week.

Boiling milk inactivates all hormones, but pasteurization does not. Except for intolerance due to the physiological loss of intestinal lactase after three years, or due to an allergy to some of the milk proteins, it would not have a contraindication, but without being an essential food, it does not add anything that is not provided by meat, fruit and vegetables. Unlike cheese and yoghurt, it is neutral or slightly acid or alkaline.

The transition from exclusive breastfeeding to semi-solid meals complementary to breastfeeding and then to general meals must be based on medical-scientific evidence. Doctors and nutrition professionals without conflicts of interest must be the active trainers of this food education and not leave it open to advertisements by processed food manufacturing companies.

Scientific evidence and uncertainties, the precautionary principle

This text is aimed at education for eating behaviours, seeking to correct empirical behaviours, creeds and myths, by means of scientific evidence on controlled studies and the knowledge of physiology and nutrition.

However the scientific evidence is not the absolute truth, it is nothing more than shrinkage of scientific uncertainty. In some cases, uncertainty dominates over the evidence and then the precautionary principle of ‘when in doubt abstain’ must be applied, following the adage of *primum non nocere* and looking for valid alternatives where the benefits do not imply greater risks.

The precautionary principle is widely applied in diagnostic and therapeutic behaviours. This same precautionary principle should also be applied to environmental exposure factors and even to the increasing number of manufactured foods, which arise from accelerated industrial development and are offered for consumption many times without sufficient evidence that they do not involve health risks.[32,33.]

Orthorexia and Anorexia

Another aspect of eating behaviour is the risk of various diseases related to the kind of food consumed, such as those referred to below.

Coeliac disease in its different manifestations is caused by the damage done by gliadin, the gluten contained in wheat and other cereals.

The risk of poisoning by heavy metals, mainly mercury, lead and arsenic that pollute the waters are present in farmed fish, or by the insecticides and fungicides with which farmers' fields are treated.

The risk from hormones, antibiotics and processed foods that are supplied to animals before their slaughter, to which is added the controversy over transgenic foods—genetically modified for greater production or resistance to herbicides and pesticides.

This has led to the need to pay special attention not to the quantity, but to the quality of food, which especially in young people, has led to behaviours that are sometimes obsessive, which leads to eliminating an increasing number of foods with consequent health risks. This new pathology in eating behaviour has been designated orthorexia, *ortho* means 'straight, correct' and *exia* means 'state'–in this case, food. In some cases, this obsession with the quality of food exposes its followers to the risk of anorexia.

Orthorexia and anorexia are both very concerning eating behaviours because not only is there a significant loss of nutrients, but the irreplaceable pleasure of eating is lost, which is one of the two pleasures in life that ensure the survival of the individual and the species and forms the basis of social integration.

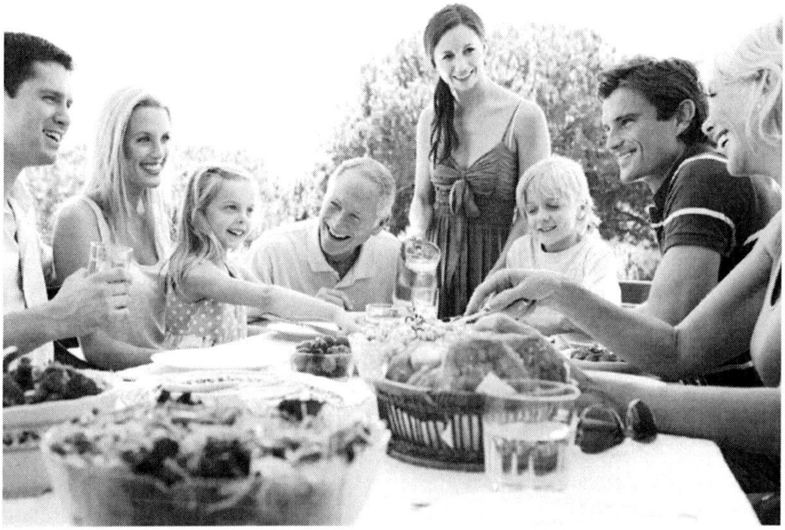

Photo 2-2: Food used for social integration

Vegetarianism and veganism

Education, mainly of particular ethical considerations, is what guides the eating behaviours of some vegetarians. The human being with its anatomical and physiological characteristics and evolutionary history, as described in Chapter 6 is omnivorous, and requires food from more than one biological kingdom. Vegans not only prohibit the consumption of meat and fish but everything of animal origin, such as milk, dairy products, eggs and honey. In addition, they will avoid using the by-products of the meat industry such as leather.

There are variants of the vegan diet, such as the raw vegan for which only raw and unprocessed foods are consumed. The diet is based on fruit, nuts, vegetables and seeds, sprouted cereals and pulses. Another variant is the frugivorous, based on fruit, nuts and seeds, including vegetables such as tomatoes and avocados. The rest of the vegetables are excluded.

The form of vegetarianism most followed in the West is that of lacto-ovo-vegetarians who include eggs and dairy in their diet. Some vegetarians and vegans, called flexitarians, allow from time to time some licenses, which with proper food education can mitigate deficiencies in some nutrients. The nutritional deficiencies of vegetarian diets, because of a lack of education and awareness, are caused by the lack of intake and poor absorption.

Vitamin B_{12} is exclusively of animal origin; it is found especially in red meat, fish and shellfish and to a lesser extent in milk and eggs. Strict vegetarians present deficiencies of this vitamin with various manifestations, such as mild neuropsychiatric disorders and mainly pernicious anaemia, and in some cases, elevated homocysteine, a coronary risk marker due to its non-conversion to methionine.

Inhabitants of India with an essentially vegetarian diet have a high incidence of coronary artery disease together with vitamin B_{12} deficiency, but without any correlation with an increase in homocysteine due to its rapid metabolization to cysteine via trans-sulfurization.[34-36.] The children of mothers who maintain a vegetarian diet during pregnancy may present neurological symptoms in the second term of life that are corrected with the supply of Vitamin B_{12}, thus avoiding sequelae damage.[37]

Vitamins B_3 or niacin and B_6 or pyridoxine and minerals, calcium, iron, zinc, iodine and magnesium are found in vegetables, but although intakes may be within normal requirements, deficiencies are frequently observed in vegetarians due to poor absorption. The malabsorption of the nutrients is due to the action of the so-called anti-nutrients, phytates, present in cereals and pulses, fibres and seeds, which act as chelators, sequestrants or binders, by forming complexes that decrease solubility and absorption. Pulses also have various oligosaccharides that cause flatulence that interfere with protein digestion.

This makes it necessary to soak the pulses six to eight hours before cooking, which should preferably be done at 130ºC in a pressure cooker, to partially inactivate the antinutrients.

Probiotics, living microorganisms incorporated into the diet, have beneficial effects on the intestinal flora and decrease the effect of antinutrients.[38] It is also known that vitamin C increases the absorption of iron because it decreases the chelating effect of the phytates on this mineral.

The possibility of incorporating phytase enzymes produced by probiotics for the dephytation of cereals and pulses is being studied by the food industry.[39-41] A widespread mistake is to consider that only meat provides protein. Nuts are an excellent source of high-quality protein, such as almonds, with a content of 19g%, walnuts 14g% and hazelnuts 12g%. Mushrooms are also an important source of protein with between 1.2 and 1.8g% in fresh mushrooms and between 19 and 35% in dried mushrooms, with all the essential amino acids.

Spinach is a vegetable with high calcium content, 210mg%, but its high content of oxalates means that it cannot be absorbed correctly. For this reason, those vegetables that have a low content of oxalates such as broccoli, Chinese kale or collards should be selected.

Vitamin C and other organic acids found in fruit and vegetables can substantially increase iron absorption and reduce the effects of phytates.

Some studies carried out on vegetarians who do not consume sources of iodine, such as iodine salt or seaweed, showed they may present a risk of iodine deficiency, as a plant-based diet is low in iodine. Foods such as soya drinks, cruciferous vegetables (broccoli, cabbage) and sweet potatoes, have substances that can sequester iodine from the body, therefore a correct combination of natural sources of iodine must be made to avoid its deficit.

Vegetable diets are generally rich in omega-6 lipid acids and may be deficient in omega-3. Diets that do not include fish, eggs or generous amounts of algae are usually low in DHA and eicosapentaenoic acid (EPA) is important for cardiovascular health and cognitive development in the infant and its preservation in the elderly. Bioconversion of linoleic acid present in plants, in EPA, is less than 10% and 3% in DHA, which are long-chain omega-3 lipid acids.

Vegetarians or vegans who do not eat a balanced diet can have low blood levels of DHA and EPA. Supplements made especially from marine microalgae or crustaceans such as krill are well-absorbed, increasing blood levels. Similarly, vitamin B_{12} supplements are necessary for strict vegetarians.

Food and Religions

In addition to eating behaviours guided by concerns over animal welfare and the environment, obsessive health concepts or purely ethical conditioning, (major factors behind vegetarianism and veganism), there are those very old eating regimes guided by the empirical precepts of religions, some of which are referred to below by their most salient characteristics.

In Judaism, the consumption of meat from land animals is allowed only if they chew the cud and have cloven hooves; the consumption of pork is not allowed despite having a cloven hoof because it does not chew the cud, nor is the consumption of rabbit meat even though it chews because it does not have a cloven hoof. Only fish with scales and fins are allowed in foods, from rivers or seas; shellfish are thus excluded.

Islam establishes some dietary rules similar to those of Judaism, such as the prohibition of the consumption of pork and a predilection for the consumption of lamb, to which is added the generous use of spices, and an absolute prohibition of alcohol.

In Christianity, there are no restrictions on various types of food, but it is established that during Lent, on Ash Wednesday and Good Friday, there must be abstinence from red meat, and fish can be consumed.

In India with its vast territory and multiplicity of social classes and ethnic groups, the diet is varied with extensive use of spices, vegetables, pulses, rice and predominantly vegetarian food, but in coastal areas, the consumption of fish and shellfish is incorporated. The most particular characteristic of Hinduism is the prohibition of the consumption of beef, as the cow is considered a sacred animal.

In the practice of Hinduism and Islam, vegetarians are frequent, so the restrictions are greater.

Generally, in religion, fasting is established for certain dates, such as Yom Kippur, Judaism's day of forgiveness, or Ramadan of Islam, which is practised for a month (the ninth of the 12 months of the Muslim calendar) from dawn to sunset and fasting in Christianity with a single normal meal during Lent, mainly during Holy Week and together with abstinence from meat except fish, on Ash Wednesday and Good Friday. Studies carried out during Ramadan, as it is the longest fast and requires strict compliance, have shown consequent metabolic changes.

A direct relationship has been observed between pre-Ramadan body mass index and a transient decrease in weight and fat mass, improvements in the lipid profile, a decrease in blood pressure, type 2 diabetes, glycated haemoglobin, adiponectin and an increase in leptin, but changes in lifestyle that accompany the Ramadan fast, such as meal times and the circadian rhythm, as markers of cardiometabolic risk, do not allow definitive conclusions attributed to fasting itself.[42-44] Fasting practices favour maintaining one of the organism's adaptive capacities practised for millions of years during evolution in times of famine.

From all the above empirically-based prescriptions, intermittent fasting can be rescued, for scientifically proven health benefits, as will be described later.

Myths and Taboos

Without religious connotations, beliefs about the benefits or risks for the health or function of various organs as well as the permissibility or rejection of certain foods without scientific grounds, vary in times and places.

For example, among the myths is the danger of combining watermelon with wine, the benefit of having bulls' testicles for strength and virility or a bean of a special class to prevent urinary stones.

Among various taboos, we mention especially what is concerned with the consumption of meat. Horse meat is not legal for consumption in the United States nor the United Kingdom, but it is accepted in several countries such as Germany, Spain, France, Italy, Russia and Japan. In Argentina, the consumption of equine meat is taboo, but the country is one of the main producers and exporters, mainly to Russia, which receives 50% of these exports. But this constitutes a marginal business; only 7% compared to beef exports.

Regional gastronomies

Some foods integrate gastronomies formerly confined to certain regions or ethnic groups or communities with particular cultures that include characteristic culinary habits. Among these foods or regional cuisines, the Mediterranean diet has been considered by epidemiological data in some respects to be especially beneficial for health, which has led to it being declared as such by UNESCO on the Intangible Cultural Heritage of Humanity list in November 2010.

As a consequence of the development of technology, especially in the food industry, transport and communications, food options have expanded dramatically since the second half of the 20th century. These regional foods have now been widely disseminated and can be consumed practically all over the world.

To this is added a large supply of processed foods, packaged drinks, some so-called energy drinks and various nutritional supplements by multinational food and pharmaceutical companies that compete with regional kitchens.

Diets

Diseases due to inborn errors of metabolism such as phenylketonuria or galactosemia, or patients in special situations such as in intensive care, with severe acute or advanced chronic kidney failure, or in certain pre and postoperative periods, or for specific diagnostic studies, require specific dietary indications. Some diets are reserved for special circumstances and times.

There are also numerous diets specifically tailored to lose weight, generally based on food restriction, mainly caloric restriction, low-calorie diets that are met for a certain time until the desired goal is achieved or are abandoned due to scant benefits.

In another sense, due to its etymology, the word diet, from the Latin *diaeta*, in turn from the Greek, *diaita*, refers to a way of life, a habit, a way of living. This is the implicit meaning of the so-called Mediterranean diet.

The Annual Review of Public Health, Annual Health Review of 2014, analyses six diets, which will be briefly referred to and which have been disseminated throughout the population, pretending to compete as among the most appropriate for the achievement of health.

Mixed-balanced

This has the orthodox proportionality in caloric contributions of the three types of macronutrients: 15% proteins, 50% carbohydrates and 35% lipids, from foods of animal and vegetable origin, without paying attention to quality depending on whether they are predominantly processed or natural. This diet is common practice in many developed or developing countries.

Low glycemic index

This has foods that do not cause sudden increases in blood glucose with strong insulin discharges leading to insulin resistance—type 2 diabetes. It may be with an increase in protein or fibre.

Special emphasis on this diet has arisen in view of the growing endemic character of diabetes.

Low in glucides

Unlike the orthodoxy that establishes the caloric intake of 15% for proteins, 50% for glucides and 35% for lipids, this diet recommends less than 45% for glucides with the consequent increase in proteins and/or lipids. In this group is 'Atkins' or the so-called keto diet and others with even greater glucides restriction favoured for the control of obesity and neurodegenerative diseases.

Obese patients treated with these diets compared to others with fat restriction show greater improvement in metabolic parameters as a decrease in glycated haemoglobin (HbA_{1c}) and low-density lipid (LDL) cholesterol.[45,46]

Low in lipids

This constitutes fewer than 20% of lipids in the caloric intake, mainly with vegetables and fruit without processed foods. In this group are vegetarians and vegans and includes flexitarians, who allow some license.

No differences were seen in the decrease in body mass index in obese children either with a low-carbohydrate or low-lipid diet.[47]

Paleolithic

Enunciated as the 'stone-age' diet in 1975 by the gastroenterologist Walter L Voegtlin[48] and also referred to as the caveman diet, or the paleo diet it is renewed and enriched with important bibliographic sources and original contributions by Eaton and Cordain among others.[49-51]

On a Darwinian evolutionary basis, it advocates a diet similar to that of our ancestors with meat, fruit and vegetables, without dairy, cereals or pulses.

The foods that our ancestors did not eat are clearly evident, such as processed foods, but meat, fruit and vegetables in the long evolutionary period of our species are different from today's meat, fruit and vegetables, due to the feed of many animals for slaughter, evolution by the selection, hybridization and even genetic engineering in the production of food of plant origin and industrialization for conservation, transport and distribution. The living conditions of our ancestors also required calories that could have been three times higher than our current needs

Mediterranean

This is characterised by the low consumption of red meat, a predominance of sea products, fish and shellfish, dried fruit, olives, olive oil, the moderate consumption of wine and a significant contribution of glucides such as starch from flour in pasta. In relation to this diet, the fact that despite its high fat consumption there is a low rate of cardiovascular and neurodegenerative diseases makes it known as 'the French paradox.' This has been attributed to the quality of the lipids, with a higher content of omega-3 polyunsaturated acids due to the consumption of olive oil, olives, nuts, seafood products and the moderate consumption of wine.

The Mediterranean diet is part of its cultural heritage, and it is not only a diet based on the main items such as fish, fruit, vegetables, nuts, olive oil, aromatic herbs as a condiment and the regular and moderate consumption of wine but lifestyle, with manual work and living a more outdoor life.

With this lifestyle combined with the Mediterranean diet, a lower incidence of chronic diseases such as diabetes, cardiovascular disease and cancer has been observed. The opposite occurs with a lifestyle of fast food and the predominance of processed foods.[52, 53]

Ketogenic

Promoted like so many others to achieve rapid weight loss, the ketogenic diet has also been referred to as more for general health benefits. For many years now, it has shown clear benefits in the control of epilepsy, especially in forms that are refractory to conventional treatment with anticonvulsant drugs.[54] Epilepsy affects approximately 1% of the population as does coeliac disease, both diseases that benefit from the exclusion of cereals. To this must be added that 8% of the population suffers from gluten sensitivity and many other patients without being epileptic present different neurological conditions that also benefit from the restriction of cereals, including autism.[55]

It is based on glucide restriction and increased lipids, with approximately 15% of calories from protein, 15% of calories from glucides and 70% of calories from lipids. This partly mimics the effect of fasting by increasing the generation of ketone bodies. A ketogenic diet for the treatment of epilepsy, under strict medical control, can provide almost 90% of calories with lipids, to which various vitamin and mineral supplements are added. The state of ketosis decreases the levels of glutamate, the main excitatory neurotransmitter, which is transformed into glutamine and gamma-aminobutyric acid (the main inhibitory neurotransmitter). It has points in common with the Atkins diet and the Paleolithic diet because it excludes cereals and pulses due to their high content of glucides.[56] It limits the consumption of fruit, preferring those that are low in glucides, such as avocados and lemons.

With the strong limitation of the referred foods, a low value in the glycemic index is also achieved.

These diets are alkaline in nature due to the richness of vegetables and the exclusion of cereals and pulses that leave strong acid residues when metabolized, but in severely ketogenic diets for the treatment of epilepsy, normal bicarbonate values are observed in the lower limits, they are mild acidosis states that lead to bone demineralization and an increased risk of kidney stones, for which it is necessary to add an alkaline supply. The ketogenic diet, in addition to facilitating weight loss, improves brain function, cognition and memory, since lipids and ketones are a quick source of energy with less production of free radicals, without a risk of oxidative stress, for which it is also anti-inflammatory.

To the above-mentioned diets is added:

Dietary approach to stop hypertension[57]

This has a predominance of vegetables, fruit, whole grains, poultry and fish and limited consumption of lean meat, skimmed milk and a restriction of sugar and salt.

As in the Mediterranean diet, vegetables, fruit, fish, poultry, dried fruit, olives and olive oil have special prevalence, with little consumption of sweets, sodium and sugary drinks. The Mediterranean diet limits red meat and includes whole wheat flour and the moderate consumption of wine.

To lose weight

Among medical prescriptions of diets for various diseases or pathological situations, diets to lose weight deserve special attention. These diets in general are based on reducing caloric intake; hypocaloric diets, but mainly attending to the quantitative aspect of calories and portions. In general lipids or glucides are strongly limited without attending to their quality. Some lipids are really unhealthy and should be avoided or strongly limited not just in treating the overweight or obese but also because they are bad for health, such as vegetable oils with a high content of omega-6 acids with pro-inflammatory action and that consumed in excess are deposited as fat. Equally bad are lipids that could be in many processed and ultra-processed foods such as trans and mega trans lipids present in margarine or derived from vegetable oils subjected to hydrogenation at high temperatures and pressure. These bad lipids cause dyslipidemias, with an increase in LDL cholesterol, a decrease in high-density lipid (HDL) cholesterol and an increased risk of cardiovascular disease.

Opposed to this are the healthy lipids with an important content of omega-3 acids, present in olive oil, avocados, walnuts and seafood. Lipids form the structure of the nervous system and favour the development in children and the preservation in adults and the elderly of cognitive capacity. The central nervous system in its composition has 60% lipids and more than half of these are made up of DHA. Many of these lipids act as neurotransmitters in neuronal interconnection.

As with lipids, some glucides are bad and should be avoided or strongly limited not only to treat or avoid being overweight or obese but because they are bad for health, as are net glucides such as sugar or high fructose corn syrup (HFCS).

Opposed to this are healthy glucides, those found in fruit and vegetables, which are energy providers together with vitamins, minerals and phytochemicals, polyphenol flavonoids and non-flavonoids that optimize vital functions. Among the glucides in fruit and vegetables are the polysaccharides that are the constituents of fibre, which slow down the absorption of glucides, thus determining a low glycemic index and preventing insulin resistance. Diets specifically aimed at losing weight without taking care or improving the state of health are not necessary or convenient.

Usual meals with meat, fish, fruit, vegetables and spices, (which is an alkaline diet with proteins, lipids and natural glucides), without processed food, without added sugar or HFCS, the limited addition of salt and without cereals or pulses, (which are reserved for occasional meals), improve health and normalize weight without especially looking for it.

Special attention must be paid to the fact that fruit in quantities of around 500 grams per day should be varied and that vegetables, in addition to using them for culinary preparations by cooking, should be raw for two or three servings combined with fruit in salads with olive oil. Meat consumed frequently, daily or three or five days a week, should be mostly cooked in water for stews or meatballs and limited to no more than one or two servings per week cooked in the oven, on the grill or fried to limit the intake of glycotoxins. Virgin apple vinegar, manufactured at home, should be included, which is the only alkaline and fermented food that will enrich the microbiota, as well as other fermented food such as beetroot kvass (beetroot extract) whose preparation, like that of virgin apple vinegar is referred to in Chapter 9.

The water provided by the aforementioned rations of fruit and vegetables, which are 80 to 90% water rich in vitamins, minerals, enzymes and phytochemicals, should be supplemented with one or two servings of vegetable soup and also with antioxidants such as two or three mugs of green tea or Yerba Mate tea instead of pure water. Sugary drinks or drinks with sweeteners are to be avoided. A sweetener that can be used for tea if desired or for some other food should be pure bee honey, thus avoiding HFCS.

Wine can also be included as a fermentation product, preferably red wine because of its higher resveratrol content, in a quantity that does not exceed 300ml for men or 200ml for women.

CHAPTER 3

FOOD EDUCATION

After the analysis and consideration of different diets, we see in the light of our current scientific knowledge, that all have some beneficial aspects for health that in some cases are shared. Other aspects are inconvenient or conflicting without the benefit of one over the other being notable.

If intense lifestyle changes are added with aerobic exercise, psychological support, stress management training and smoking cessation, a clear improvement is observed in the evolution of coronary arteriosclerosis with a decrease in coronary stenosis; 4.5% per year and 7.9% at five years compared to worsening in the control group, which showed an increase in stenosis of 2.3% per year and 11.3% at five years.[58]

Food education allows us to choose various natural foods from the three biological kingdoms, animal, plant and fungal, combined with knowing the best way to prepare, combine and ingest nutrients. Proteins of high biological value (meat, eggs, fish and mushrooms) good quality lipids (olive oil, avocado, nuts, coconut and cocoa butter and fish) and natural glucides (fruit, vegetables and honey) are foods that when eaten in a variety also provide the minerals, vitamins and phytochemicals essential for health.

Experimental laboratory studies with animals and clinical and epidemiological observations of patients and population groups with prolonged follow-ups and controls in full development over several years have provided scientific evidence on the synergistic effects of micronutrients and phytochemicals of fruit and vegetables that optimize vital functions.

To this is added, based on current scientific knowledge, the use of spices, not only as condiments but also for taking advantage of their beneficial effects for the preservation of health and the prevention of various diseases.

The proper balance between omega-6 and omega-3 lipid acids, essential for anti-inflammatory and antithrombotic actions and the control of oxidative stress are important participants in the prevention and treatment of an increasing number of diseases: the increase and modulation of immunological defences, anticancer action, preservation of molecular structures of proteins and nucleic acids for cellular integrity and metabolic functions, prevention of bacterial and viral infections, arteriosclerosis, autoimmune, metabolic and neurodegenerative diseases.

Compounds belonging to groups of phytochemicals such as flavonoid and non-flavonoid polyphenols, lycopene, lignans and squalene, have numerous beneficial properties for health such as powerful antioxidant action, and many of these have anti-cancer properties or stimulating enzymes for the inactivation of xenobiotics. Compounds of the animal kingdom especially from seafood, such as long-chain lipid acids, docosahexaenoic, arachidonic and eicosapentaenoic, as we have already said, favour cognitive development during infancy and preserve mental deterioration in senescence, while an adequate balance between omega-6 and omega-3 lipid acids is essential for anti-inflammatory and antithrombotic actions.

The numerous knowledge and theories to understand what, why and to what extent certain foods are essential for our usual meals and how they should be ingested and at the same time understand which and why there are foods that are not essential and involve health risks when they are ingested regularly, is the central axis for the achievement of healthy eating behaviour.

Although any orientation or set of directives on food is liable to be called a diet, the contents of this book are not intended in any way to be included in that heading.

Food education intends to achieve lifelong behaviours to preserve health and prevent disease in an ethical framework, by promoting its good repercussions on the family and society.

Food education must start in childhood, which has a multiplier effect in the future, with natural foods varying in colour and consistency; fruit, vegetables, eggs and meat given during the first years of life, complementing lactation.

With porridge, yellow pumpkin and carrot, white sweet potato, green chard and spinach, with added meat and egg supplied with a teaspoon, it is common to hear from mothers the phrase: "it does not eat me" meaning they take it personally when the food is rejected. In recent years it is common to make suitable foods available to children so that they can choose without trying to impose anything on them and provoke rejection. This should be done with the direct advice of a paediatrician or nutritionist versed in the subject. The baby-lead weaning or self-regulated meals complementary to breastfeeding for the incorporation of solid foods is the method by which the child, from six months old, takes food placed at their fingertips so that they can choose, before the watchfulness of their parents without trying to impose on them and provoke rejection. The food should be soft, 2 or 3cm in size, such as pieces of ripe banana, tomato, avocado or cooked pumpkin, sweet potato, carrot, apple, egg or pieces of meat or chicken cut transversely. Hard foods such as dried cherries, walnuts, almonds, hazelnuts or whole grapes should not be placed within reach and parents should always be close to the child to avoid choking.

Juice should not be given. Children should be accustomed to chewing soft food with their gums and get used to their natural tastes without added sugar.

Eating behaviour according to cultural, social, economic and climatic determinants that make it elastic, flexible and adaptable to circumstances and places, but within certain limits, do not imply loss of freedom, since by minimizing risks, it simply becomes a responsible exercise.

Vegetables, fruit, meat, eggs, mushrooms, in a subtle order of priorities, and spices, are 'biological virtues' worth the metaphor, for our organism. If we also avoid a sedentary lifestyle and live in balance with the natural and social environment, the achievement of health is highly probable, which is not just the absence of disease but also good physical, mental and social well-being.

It is good to become familiar with the elements of the chemical structure of our food.

We classify food into three large groups: lipids, glucides and proteins.

Among its multiple functions, we can show that lipids are the main source of energy reserve in animals and are structural components, fundamental in cell membranes and the nervous system. Glucides allow a rapid availability of energy and proteins mainly constitute the structure of cells and tissues and regulate vital functions with enzymatic actions.

Lipids

Lipids are generally called fats and therefore the basic constituents of these foods are called fatty acids. It would be more correct to call them lipid acids.

Solid lipids at room temperature, such as those of animal origin, are properly called fats and liquid lipids, such as those of vegetable origin, are oils. We say, for example, subcutaneous fat and olive oil. However, two vegetable lipids are solid in their natural state at room temperature; the lipids of cocoa and coconut, and are called cocoa butter and coconut butter, which melt at 37°C, transforming into oils. In the case of cocoa butter, a basic constituent of chocolate, we can see how it easily liquefies in the mouth.

Since the 1950s, the risk of cardiovascular disease with alterations in the plasma lipid profile, elevations of triglycerides and cholesterol at the expense of *LDL* the so-called 'bad' cholesterol, which is bad only when it is oxidized, has been associated with the consumption of fats. The bad reputation of fats was attributed not only to the fact that they contain cholesterol but also to the chemical structure of many of their acids, which are saturated. This led to showing the virtues of cholesterol-free lipids, vegetable oils and especially those unsaturated, which are currently under review.

Saturated and unsaturated lipid acids

Lipid acids are made up of chains of variable lengths of carbon atoms linked together by bonds that can be of two kinds: single bonds that make *saturated lipid acids* and double bonds that make *unsaturated lipid acids*.

The lipid acids that have all their carbons joined by single bonds are saturated.

The lipid acids that have one or more of their carbons linked by double bonds are unsaturated and are monounsaturated or polyunsaturated depending on whether they have one or more double bond in their chains.

In carbon atoms, in addition to the bonds that join them together, other bonds join them to hydrogen atoms, except the last carbon on the right attached to O and hydroxyl (OH), which form the carboxyl (COOH) acid end. The first carbon in the chain on the left, with three H, forms the methyl (CH_3) alkaline end.

Simple links

```
 |   |
- C - C-
 |   |
```

Double links

```
  |     |
— C  =  C —
```

A short-chain of four-carbon lipid acid is *butyric acid*, which is referred to as 4:0. This means that it has four carbons joined together by single bonds; the 0 denotes that there is no double bond, so it is said to be a saturated lipid acid.

```
    H   H   H   O
    |   |   |   |
H - C - C - C - C - OH
    |   |   |
    H   H   H
```

Butyric acid

Since we are dealing with *butyric acid,* it is appropriate to note that it is very good for health, as it is the main nutrient of the intestinal cell or enterocyte, which preserves the integrity and length of the *intestinal villi.* This allows for the adequate absorption of nutrients, the appropriate defence mechanisms by a mechanical barrier and by immunological mechanisms against infections and the passage of toxins from the intestinal lumen. This is an example that not all saturated lipid acids are 'bad', as has been widely reported.

Butyric acid is mostly not found in food, except in small amounts in some fats such as butter. It is produced by the intestinal bacterial flora from the fermentation of the fibre present in vegetables and fruit. For this and many other actions, vegetables and fruit should always be an important part of our usual meals, which should include a minimum of two or three servings a day.

Another saturated lipid acid is palmitic acid, a long chain with 16 carbons, (16:0) present, especially in fats, of animal origin.

Palmitic acid is synthesized in the body and as a physiological action, it should be noted that from it, the human body can synthesize the other lipid acids it requires, with the exception of essential lipid acids, so-called because the body cannot synthesize them and they must come from food. *Essential lipid acids* are linoleic and linolenic acid. Excessive consumption of saturated lipid acids, the most common palmitic acid, has harmful effects on health, mainly cardiovascular disease, to which they have been attributed and this is currently under review.

Saturated lipid reconsideration

Saturated lipid acids are butyric, stearic, lauric and palmitic.

Unsaturated lipids are unstable; they are oxidized by air, light and heat. Of the polyunsaturates, the monounsaturated ones are preferable. On the other hand, the benefits of lipids, as they are present in natural foods, are currently highlighted. Modern research techniques on the different lipid components and their significance in the risk of cardiovascular disease may incorporate new contributions aimed at clarifying a topic that is still a matter of controversy.[59] The main source of excessive consumption of saturated lipids is not natural foods, but processed foods. To reduce the risk of cardiovascular disease and implicit stroke, it is beneficial to limit the consumption of refined glucides, especially processed foods containing margarine, and lose weight where necessary.

Concerning the increased risk of cardiovascular disease due to an increase in saturated fats and a decrease in polyunsaturated fats, prospective epidemiological studies have not consistently shown this, and some of the results are even contradictory.[60-65] The term saturated fat is generally incorrect; lipids are made up of a variable number of lipid acids, some saturated and others unsaturated, and these are mono or polyunsaturated. Replacing saturated lípids with mono and polyunsaturated lowers LDL and HDL, but polyunsaturated lipid acids are more unstable and susceptible to oxidation. The replacement of foods with saturated lipids is usually done with a higher glucides intake, in particular, refined ones can produce atherogenic dyslipidemias with increased triglycerides.

This favours the production of atheroma plaques in the vascular walls, which increases rigidity and decreases the calibre of vascular circulation. Less tissue irrigation can cause cell death, necrosis and ischemic infarction. Insulin resistance and obesity are associated with dyslipidemia.[66-68]

What is really necessary to reduce the risk of cardiovascular disease, evidently related to weight gain and obesity, is education about food that encourages increased consumption of vegetables and fruit for the highest fibre intake that this implies, and avoiding a disproportionate intake of meat, fish, dairy products, processed foods, salt, sugar and alcohol and correcting smoking and sedentary lifestyles.[69]

Olive oil, butter and coconut butter are the best ingredients for cooking, not sunflower or corn oil, not only because of their low content of omega-3 and high of omega-6 but because when frying, the smoking point is lower than that of olive oil, which has a higher than necessary smoking point during frying, which avoids the generation of carcinogenic products.

The so-called Mediterranean paradox or French paradox proposes an explanation for the reduced incidence of cardiovascular disease in Mediterranean countries, despite their high proportion of dietary lipids, olive oil and moderate consumption of wine (analyzed in detail later). In these countries, most of the lipids come from olive oil, which provides oleic acid as a fundamental lipid acid. Traditionally it has been consumed unrefined; it is the so-called *virgin olive oil*, which provides various phytochemicals with antioxidant properties, which gives an additional protective role against oxidative stress and lipid peroxidation.

Oleic acid (octadecaenoic; C18: 1n-9) is the fundamental dietary representative of monounsaturated lipid acids.

Eicosanoids with vasodilator and antiplatelet activity are derived from oleic acid. At the lipid level, it causes a reduction in triglycerides, total cholesterol and LDL, as well as its oxidation, with the added benefit of being one of the few known substances capable of inducing the elevation of HDL.

Due to the bad, albeit unjustified reputation of fats, *margarine* derived from vegetable oils and therefore cholesterol-free was wrongly considered to be a healthier option than butter, which is of animal origin. Margarine was obtained by the food industry in the 1920s from vegetable oils by hydrogenation processes at high temperatures and under pressure. Margarine wrongly came to be preferred over butter for being more resistant to rooting and oxidation and was, therefore, easier to preserve. Over time it was seen that this actually had economic benefits for producers, due to better preservation and easier transport than vegetable oils, but it has serious health implications due to the generation of *trans* fats. For several years now, it has been known that trans fats are more dangerous than saturated fats because are strongly associated with the risk of cardiovascular disease. They not only increase the so-called bad cholesterol or LDL but, unlike saturated fats, they lower the 'good' cholesterol, or HDL.[70,71]

Forms cis and trans

Unsaturated lipid acids are mono or polyunsaturated depending on whether they have one or more double bonds. All unsaturated lipid acids are long-chain, with more than 10 carbons. Take for example only the part of the chain of an unsaturated lipid acid where the double bond is, if the two hydrogens are on the same side it is the *cis* form and if they are on opposite sides, it is the *trans* form.

Form cis

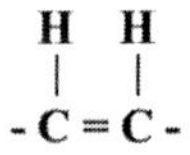

Form trans

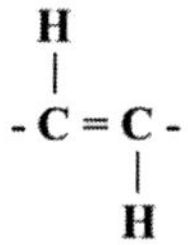

In the process of the hydrogenation of vegetable oils to obtain margarine, it is common for hydrogens of carbons with double bonds to change the cis position for the transposition. These lipids are called trans and they can represent up to 40% of total lipids. Trans lipid acids are also present in foods from ruminant, polygastric animals, produced by bacterial action, but they do not exceed 3 or 4% of the total. In human food, the main source of trans lipids comes from hydrogenated vegetable oils and margarine present in various products, such as cereal bars or biscuits, where they can represent between 10 and 30% of total lipids. The trans lipids determine the release by some cells of substances that act on other cells, neighbouring or distant substances called cytokines, which in this case as IL6, tumour necrosis factor-alpha (TNFα) and C-reactive protein (CRP) have pro-inflammatory actions and favour the production of thrombi, clots adhered to the vascular walls that obstruct blood circulation.[72,73]

Trans fats cross the placenta and are present in milk during lactation and could affect the pre and postnatal development and growth of a child.[74-76] This has led to restricting the inclusion of trans fats in foods as much as possible.

In response to this, the industry has sought to minimize the presence of trans fats in margarine by modifying the hydrogenation process and adding water, emulsifiers, flavourings, preservatives, vitamins, salt, and sometimes milk and intensely shaking products to achieve water and oil emulsions stabilized by fat crystals.[77, 78] In several countries, there is legislation in this regard, and it is advisable to read the food labelling where the trans-fat content of the product appears. The WHO and the FAO recommend fewer than 1% of calories in the diet from trans fats. This means for consumption of 2000 calories a day, which may be typical for a 70kg adult, no more than 2g of trans fat per day.

Apart from trans fats present in margarine, let us assume that margarine is made from vegetable oils, from seeds such as sunflower, corn or soya. These oils are not recommended for consumption in the usual diet, as they all have a low or very low content of omega-3 lipid acids and a high content of omega-6 lipid acids. Therefore, they have a pro-inflammatory action, different from olive oil that is not from the seed but the fruit, (olives), with a high content of omega-3 lipid acids with anti-inflammatory action, which is why they should be the ones commonly consumed.

Vegetable oils and butter

Vegetable oils most commonly used both in the kitchen and at the table are those from sunflower and corn seeds; they are made up of polyunsaturated fatty acids. For this reason, they are more unstable and more susceptible to damage by oxidation in the face of heat and light. In addition, the high ratio of omega-6/omega-3 is much higher than convenient, therefore they have pro-inflammatory action. Vegetable oils are not recommended to season our meals or to cook with.

The processed food industry, through the hyper hydrogenation of vegetable oils, achieved their solidification, margarine, which as we said is more resistant to going rancid and easier to transport. Later it was found that margarine, because of its trans fats content, is more harmful to health than saturated fats.

Omega-6 and omega-3 lipid acids

The designation of lipid acids as *omega-6 or omega-3* comes from the Greek, which is read from right to left, where the first letter on the right of the alphabet is alpha and the last letter on the left is omega.

Omega-6 for example means that counting from the first carbon on the left, the omega end, on carbon-6 there is a double bond. Referring to a long chain monounsaturated lipid acid with a double bond in carbon 9, the oleic acid is represented as 18:1 n-9. Referring to long-chain polyunsaturated lipid acids, the pro-inflammatory linoleic acid, with 18 carbons and two double bonds in carbon 6 and 9 is represented as 18:2 n-6,9. The anti-inflammatory linolenic acid with three double bonds in carbons 3,6 and 9, is represented as 18:3 n-3, 6, 9.

We must also represent the important long-chain lipid acids, the pro-inflammatory omega-6 alpha-linolenic, 20:4 n-6,9,12,15 and the anti-inflammatory omega-3 *EPA*, 20:5 n-3,6,9,12,15 and *DHA*, 22:6 n-3, 9,12,15,18.

The body's inflammatory response is a physiological process of defence against various toxins, trauma, infections and damage to certain organs or tissues, and is aimed at limiting and neutralizing that damage, but it must only remain in place for as long as necessary. The problem arises when the inflammatory response becomes a generalized and permanent process, a state of chronic inflammation. This is a promoter of diabetes, obesity, cardiovascular disease, rheumatoid arthritis and even cancer. A balance is necessary, as it is risky to almost nullify the inflammatory reaction, but an excessive and persistent inflammatory reaction is a conditioning and aggravating factor of many diseases.

Index omega-6/omega-3

In a diet, there must be a balance between pro-inflammatory and anti-inflammatory agents, between omega-6 and omega-3 lipid acids.

Arachidonic acid is a pro-inflammatory factor and an excess of this is not healthy. Hence, AA food sources such as meat, (beef, pork, goat, poultry etc.), or eggs, must be balanced with foods that provide omega-3 such as fish, especially salmon, tuna, sardines or seafood at least two times a week, and walnuts, which have an omega-6/omega-3 index of 5.

An omega-6/omega-3 index close to 10 is considered optimal; 10 omega-6 to 1 omega-3. In the most common Western diets, this index is high, around 20 or 30.

With regard to different oils, sunflower oil has practically no omega-3, to give a figure it can be said that the omega-6/omega-3 index is 200 or 300, and in corn oil, it is 30, both from the oil of the seeds.

Extra virgin olive oil, which is not from the seed but the fruit, (olives), has an omega 6-/omega-3 index of 12. Extra virgin olive oil should be preferred for both culinary and domestic use. Its main lipid acid is oleic acid, and it also has various phytochemicals, including phenolic compounds that protect against oxidative stress and lipid peroxidation. From oleic acid, vasodilator eicosanoids with antiplatelet action are derived, they reduce triglycerides, total cholesterol and LDL and protect it from oxidation and are one of the few substances that increase HDL.

Flax oil has an extremely low omega-6/omega-3 index of 0.2, it is strongly anti-inflammatory, and it can be used almost as a medicine against excessive inflammatory processes, but it is not for regular nutrition because the body exerts inflammation as a reaction to overcome different processes.

Vegetable oils with a high omega-6/omega-3 index are responsible for systemic inflammatory processes and the alteration of cell membranes and chromosomal damage, also increasing triglycerides. In addition, due to the refinement process to which they are subjected, they suffer the oxidation of polyunsaturated lipid acids generating free radicals and mutations that make them even more harmful, which is why they are called *megatrans*. Megatrans lipids cause alterations in endothelial functions with a decrease in the arterial dilation capacity, which does not exceed 1% compared to the normal 7%, which is the cause of heart attacks.[79]

Coconut oil contains medium-chain lipid acids, which cross cell membranes and provide energy, they do not go to fat deposits. Coconut oil is very resistant to oxidation, unlike olive oil. Among its lipid acids that are saturated, lauric is antibacterial.

Among the vegetable oils, some rape-seed oil is called *canola oil.* Canola comes from "Canadian oil low acid", referring to the erucic acid contained in rape seed, and that is the oil used for industrial machines as a lubricant as it has concentrations the same as found in the seeds, up to 30 and 40% of the total lipids. *Erucic acid* produces lipidosis and fibrosis of the myocardium, with decreased contractility. By isothiocyanates it binds to iodine and reduces thyroxine; it is goitrogenic. For culinary use, the concentration of this acid should not be more than 2%. It is advisable to note the concentration of erucic acid on the labelling of commercial containers.

When talking about the omega-3 content of various foods, the difference between omega-3 of vegetable origin and those of animal origin must be highlighted. Of plant origin, is the 18-carbon long-chain alfa linolenic acid, from which very long-chain 20 and 22carbons are derived by hepatic metabolization, such as EPA and DHA, but only in a small fraction, 1 to 3%.

Of animal origin, in the fat of marine animals, fish, shellfish and crustaceans, the very long-chain EPA and DHA are already present. Especially recommended are small fish such as sardines and anchovies. These organisms, due to their shorter life span have less accumulation of toxins that pollute marine waters, such as mercury. Larger fish such as tuna and salmon are available in many countries from sea farms.

EPA and DHA especially promote cognitive and visual development in childhood and are also found in human milk, but not in cow's milk. These acids are also important for the preservation of cognitive abilities in adult life and senescence. A relationship has also been observed between the intake of fish or shellfish and the lower incidence of depression.[80,81] EPA and DHA showed beneficial effects on cardiovascular health, decreased platelet aggregation and the risk of atrial fibrillation, among other cardiovascular hemodynamic effects.[82] Diets rich in omega-3 lipidic acids have a renal protective effect in diabetes.[83] Foods that have indicated their composition show their omega-3 content but not the type of omega-3, which does not allow us to deduce their true nutritional value.

Glucides

Glucides, a term derived from the Greek meaning 'sweet', are also called saccharides and misnamed *carbohydrates*, are molecules of carbon, hydrogen and oxygen. Their general formula is presented as $C_n\ (H_2O)_n$.

The suffix n is the number of atoms, or molecules varying according to their complexity. Due to this way of representing the general formula of these substances, the name carbohydrates arose. That designation is inappropriate, as they are not hydrated carbon atoms nor linked to water molecules. The unions, as is typical in organic chemistry, are covalent bonds.

Covalent bonds occur between elements with little or no difference in electrical charges, where the atoms bond together by sharing electrons. These bonds are difficult to break and store large amounts of energy that is released by oxidation.

The designation of sugars applies only to monosaccharides and disaccharides, and the singular refers to purified sucrose or table sugar.

Simple and complex

According to the number of molecules that make them, those with up to 10 molecules are referred to as simple and those with more than 10 molecules, are as complex.

Simple glucides are monosaccharides, disaccharides and oligosaccharides, which have between 3 and 9 molecules.

Complex glucides are those with 10 or more, up to hundreds or thousands of molecules.

Monosaccharides

Depending on the number of carbon atoms in a molecule, ranging from three to seven, they are triose, tetrose, pentoses, hexoses or heptoses. Only the most important in physiology and nutrition will be mentioned. These are formed by a chain of six carbons; they are hexoses:

Glucose, fructose and galactose

- Glucose, dextrose; blood sugar. Two glucose molecules make the disaccharide maltose or malt sugar, together with galactose it integrates the disaccharide lactose, which is milk sugar and together with fructose, it makes the disaccharide sucrose, or common sugar, from sugar cane.

- Fructose, or levulose; fruit sugar. Fructose and glucose make the disaccharide sucrose, or common sugar, from sugar cane.
- Galactose, with glucose integrates the disaccharide lactose, which is milk sugar.

Monosaccharides do not require digestion; they are absorbed directly into the blood.

Glucose

Glucose is the most abundant organic compound and the primary source of energy.

The main glucose consumers in the body are the muscles and fat and they need insulin, secreted by the pancreas, to help it enter the cell and be metabolized. In insulin resistance or deficiency, type 2 or type 1 diabetes respectively, the muscles and fat cannot use it and there is more glucose available for the other tissues whose cells incorporate it directly, without insulin requirement. The excess glucose activates the enzyme aldose reductase which transforms glucose into fructose.

Fructose

Fructose, like glucose, is a hexose. For several years now, high fructose corn syrup (HFCS) has largely replaced common sugar or sucrose in processed foods. This has considerably increased fructose consumption, which is not recommended due to its rapid intracellular entry since it does not require insulin, with pathogenic effects that will be exposed when developing the topic of glycation later on. In addition, its metabolism produces uric acid, whose inflammatory action can cause particular forms of arthritis, a disease called gout. The concentration of fructose in the blood reaches only 1% of glycemia due to its rapid intracellular entry.

Galactose

With glucose, galactose integrates the disaccharide lactose or milk sugar, which is a natural and optimal food during the lactation period and specific for each species. Breastfeeding therefore must be exclusive for the first six months from birth, supplemented thereafter with semi-solid foods to extend to no less than nine months, and as far as possible until the second year of life, that is to say throughout early childhood.

Disaccharides: Maltose, Sucrose and Lactose

- *Maltose* or malt sugar is made up of two glucose molecules.
- *Sucros*e or cane sugar is made up of glucose and fructose.
- *Lactose* or milk sugar is made up of glucose and galactose.

Disaccharides require digestion by the action of enzymes present in the intestinal villi that release the respective monosaccharides. These enzymes are:

- *Maltase* that digests maltose, releasing two glucose molecules.
- *Sucrase* that digests sucrose, releasing one molecule of glucose and another of fructose.
- *Lactase* that digests lactose, releasing one molecule of glucose and another of galactose.

This digestion is easy, and the rapid absorption of monosaccharides allows an immediate availability of energy.

The disaccharide sucrose is commonly known as sugar, or table sugar because it is the most commonly used sweetener.

Oligosaccharides

Formed by the union of between 3 and 9 monosaccharides:

- *Raffinose* (trisaccharide, with galactose, fructose and glucose).
- *Stachyose* (tetrasaccharide, with two galactoses, fructose and glucose).
- *Verbascosa* (pentasaccharide, with three galactoses, fructose and glucose).

Polysaccharides

Made up of chains of 10 to hundreds of thousands of monosaccharides, they are reserve glucides like starch or inulin, or structural glucids like pectin or cellulose.

The reserve *polysaccharides*, starch and inulin in the plant kingdom, formed by chains of glucose or fructose respectively, are equivalent to glycogen in the animal kingdom, but glycogen is more rapidly metabolized, which is appropriate given the more active animal metabolism.

The starch in tubers, tuberous roots and grains can supply plants with an energy source for several days. Hepatic glycogen in animals maintains fasting blood glucose for only six hours; the main energy reserves in animals are lipids.

Most cells have polysaccharides on their surface for protection and recognition, as the major histocompatibility complex.

The structure of polysaccharides, mainly cellulose, a fibre component, in the membranes of plant and fungal cells gives them a hydrostatic skeleton. Chitin is the basis of the arthropod exoskeleton and is part of the cell walls of fungi.

- Starch is a glucose polymer with two compounds, 25 to 30% amylose with a helical structure and 70 to 75% amylopectin with a branched structure.
- Inulin, a fructose polymer, is a fructosan or fructan.
- Fructo-oligosaccharides are oligo-fructans.

Starch

Starch, which is formed by long chains of glucose, is a polymer of glucose and is difficult to digest, but cooking produces smaller chains, which facilitates its digestion and absorption.

The great stability of starch, has, since palaeontological times, provided interesting contributions to the diets of our ancestors.

Homo sapiens have amylase in the salivary glands and pancreas in an amount three times higher than that observed in the chimpanzee. This allows them to survive in times of meat and fruit shortages.

Inulin

Inulin, like starch, is an energy reserve polysaccharide in vegetables. It is soluble fibre and gives rise to fructo-oligosaccharides.

Fructo-oligosaccharides. Soluble fibre

Fructo-oligosaccharides are made up of 10 to 20 fructose monomers, some with an initial glucose molecule: kestose, nystose, inulotriose, inulotetrose, bifurcose, inulobiose and fructosylinestrose.

Natural fructo-oligosaccharides are found especially in chicory, garlic, onions and asparagus and have been obtained industrially from chicory, by degradation of inulin or by synthesis from sucrose by transfructosylation.

Starch, inulin, glycogen and fructo-oligosaccharides act as depot carbohydrates.

They have been recommended as a substitute for sugar due to their very low caloric value, 1 to 2.8 kcal/g. with 30 to 50% of the sweetening power of sugar.

In the diet, they behave like a soluble fibre of small molecular weight. They favour the development of normal intestinal bacterial flora, which is why they are referred to as prebiotics and hinder the development of pathogenic bacteria such as salmonellae and shigella.[84-86]

As they are not digested by salivary or intestinal amylase, they reach the large intestine where they are degraded by the bacterial flora, generating short-chain lipid acids, including butyric acid, a nutrient of the intestinal epithelium. In this fermentation process, acidity increases and intestinal pH decreases, this favours the absorption of calcium and magnesium.[87,88]

All the stated benefits of fructo-oligosaccharides together with other indigestible polysaccharides, soluble and insoluble fibres, allow them to be considered functional foods.

Glycemic index and glycemic load

In addition to the chemical classification of glucides, from a nutritional point of view, their classification and the foods that contain them according to their *glycemic index* (GI) are important. GI is the degree of increase in blood glucose observed within two hours after ingestion. The value of 100 corresponding to glucose is considered a reference. It is also important to take into account the *glycemic load* (GL) that is the content of glucid.

The GL is what really gives significance to the GI, that is, its impact on blood glucose. It does not make sense to take into account the GI of meat due to its low glucid content, that is, due to the low GL. Numerous prospective studies show that a habitual diet where high GL predominates and consequently strong and repeated insulin discharges promotes being weight gain, obesity, type 2 diabetes, cardiovascular disease, certain types of cancer and inflammatory processes that are important participants of these and other diseases.

Fruit and vegetables have a low GI, generally between 20 and 50 due to the fibre content that slows down the absorption of glucides and due to their high water content of 80 to 95%, consequently creating a low GL. This determines that even an abundant intake of fruit and vegetables, in addition to low caloric intake, does not determine significant increases in blood glucose.

Foods made with refined grains such as cereal flours, for example, pasta or white bread, have a high GI, generally between 50 and 70 partially due to their low water content. The habitual and abundant ingestion of these foods determines strong and significant peaks of glycemia and important caloric contributions that lead to weight gain and obesity.[89]

The highest GI present in dense foods, such as white bread is also because they do not have fibre which slows the absorption of glucides. Due to low GI and low GL, the intake of vegetables and fruit, with high nutritional density and low caloric density, should be part of our usual meals with no less than 2 or 3 servings daily. With its ingestion, strong insulin discharges are not produced.

Contrary to this, there are processed foods with high GI and high GL due to sugar or fructose syrup. Pastries, bread and pasta are foods with an especially high caloric density and low nutritional density.

Due to the content not only of net glucides but also of lipids, such as margarine or vegetable oils such as sunflower or corn, together with a sedentary lifestyle, they favour the development of hepatic steatosis, a fatty liver, a higher incidence of hypercholesterolemia, colorectal and breast cancer, cataracts in old age, chronic kidney disease, type 2 diabetes and neurological disorders.

In recent years, even Alzheimer's disease has been related to this pathogenesis,[90] as has chronic kidney failure in adults with no history of kidney disease or diabetes.[91]

The GI varies for the same food according to its preparation, for example with carrots and raw beetroot the GI is 30, but when cooked it is 85 and 60 respectively.

Apart from vegetables, processed foods such as farinaceous (bread and pasta) which abound in the Mediterranean diet, where cooking increases digestibility and absorption, have a high GI of 60 and 100 respectively. Likewise, in white rice, due to its starch content, the GI of 65, after cooking, rises to 95. Like high and low extremes of GI, we can take corn syrup with 110 and pumpkin, onion or fruit with 15.

Below we can see the GI of common foods. Table 3-1.

Glycemic index

Breads and pastries		**Legumes 26 to 39**	
Baguette	95	Soya	18
Doughnuts	76	Peanuts	14
White bread	73		
Wholewheat bread	51		
Fruit		**Vegetables**	
Pineapple	58	Beetroot	64
Potato	50	Carrot	30
Apricot	57		
Kiwi	53		
Banana	52		
Grape	46		
Orange	42		
Pear	38		
Apple	38		
Rice			
Low amylase	83-88	White	64
High amylose	56	Whole grain	34
Sugar and substitutes			
Cherry	72	Glucose	99
Sucrose	68	Honey	55
Fructose	19	Xylitol	8
Pasta			
Noodles	47	Macaroni	47
Spaghetti	38		

Table 3-1
Source: Wikipedia, Glycemic index[92, 93].

Sugar

Common sugar or table *sugar* is the sucrose extracted by industrial procedures mainly from sugar cane and it is purified until granules, or a white powder is obtained.

Cane juice obtained by pressing contains sucrose, a disaccharide formed by glucose and fructose, plus fibre, which are complex glucides, dextrin as a polysaccharide and raffinose as an oligosaccharide. It also contains B vitamins and minerals such as potassium, iron, magnesium, manganese and calcium.

Sugar cane juice, with partial loss of water by cooking, gives rise to molasses. Cooking leads to loss of water until obtaining a powder. Barbados sugar, or Muscovado sugar, molasses and Muscovado sugar retain to a variable degree the original properties of cane juice.

White or table sugar is obtained by filtration to remove fibre or bagasse and is clarified with sulfur dioxide and lime. After cooking and filtering, infusorium earth and phosphoric acid are added, discarding solid waste or cachaça. After boiling and evaporation in vacuo, the sucrose crystallizes. The crystals are bleached with ultramarine blue.

Black sugar results from treating banked sugar with molasses extract obtained by the fermentation of corn or barley.

The industrial process for obtaining sugar eliminates complex glucides, vitamins and minerals. This reduces the nutritional value to the exclusive caloric contribution of sucrose, an easily digestible and rapidly absorbed disaccharide with a high GI. Consumption of sugar should be reduced to a minimum or even avoided, due to the damage of high GI and glycation produced on proteins, lipids and nucleic acids, with an alteration of mitochondrial metabolism causing important diseases, or even carcinogenic conditions.

Likewise, sugar is to be avoided in all diets for weight reduction, which is mainly the reason for the widespread use of synthetic sweeteners, which is not recommended either.

Sweeteners

Synthetic *sweeteners* are derived from the chemical industry, such as *saccharin*, obtained from petroleum derivatives, *sucralose* obtained by halogenating sucrose, *aspartame* or *acesulfame.* Other sweeteners are *xylitol,* which is a polyol and *stevia*, which is a natural sweetener of plant origin. Both deserve special consideration other than synthetic sweeteners. The use of synthetic sweeteners as part of weight-loss diets is not recommended. The sweetening action perceived in the taste buds determines an anticipatory reaction of insulin discharge by the pancreas which, if there is no glucid intake, determines a drop in blood glucose with an anorexigenic effect, which can increase caloric intake. The regular use of synthetic sweeteners should also be avoided because they affect the development of intestinal bacterial flora.[94]

Maximum permissible doses of synthetic sweeteners are higher than would be used normally in the home, but it should be noted that they are generously incorporated in diet products, jams, sweets, pastries and beverages.

Cyclamates have been banned in the United States since 1970 due to controversy surrounding the carcinogenic effect observed in rats, although at doses 100 times higher than those used as a sweetener. Also, saccharin has been linked to bladder cancer in rats.

Aspartame has the amino acid phenylalanine in its composition, which can indirectly increase appetite by reducing the production of serotonin, which has an anorectic action and also slows down metabolism.[95,96]All these products have a sweetening effect 40 to 200 times higher than table sugar.

Allergic reactions with itching, conjunctival irritation, sneezing and nasal congestion can be observed with any of these products.

Xylitol has no particular adverse effects.

Stevia, extracted from the leaves of the stevia rebaudiana plant, a shrub native to northern Paraguay and southern Brazil, has been used for centuries as a sweetener. For decades it has also been used as a hypotensive in Brazil. Currently, 40% of stevia production is consumed in Japan. Its action as a sweetener is 300 times greater than that of table sugar and it has iron, zinc, phosphorus, calcium, potassium and vitamins A and C. In experimental animals, cell cultures and humans with controlled studies, the metabolic actions of its active principles have been verified.

Glycosides, stevioside and rebaudioside with therapeutic implications and doses of 200 to 2000mg/kg, three times a day lack toxic effects and are without adverse reactions even during pregnancy. After ingestion and hydrolyzation by the intestinal microflora, they are absorbed to be metabolized in the liver with a protective action on its parenchyma. Excretion occurs through faecal matter and urine.

Stevioside has a hypotensive effect, increases insulin sensitivity, helps to control glycemia and inhibits gluconeogenesis without causing hypoglycemia. It exerts antioxidant and anti-inflammatory actions and attenuates metabolic syndrome. Metabolic parameters were observed in addition to the reduction in blood glucose and improvement in the homeostasis model assessment index (HOMA), a decrease in inflammatory markers such as interleukin 6 and tumour necrosis factor-alpha. They reduce hypercholesterolemia, with a decrease in LDL and the risk of cardiovascular disease and atherogenesis. Thus, they have therapeutic implications in the control of obesity and consequently, in metabolic syndrome.[97]They have also shown benefits in the evolutionary control of chronic kidney failure and prevention of cardiovascular disease.

Clinical tests in patients with chronic renal failure show a decrease in microalbuminuria and serum levels of creatinine, glycemia and uric acid.[98] Unfortunately, products on the market labelled as stevia also have various sweeteners as ingredients such as sucrose, sucralose or acesulfame.

Honey

Produced from the nectar of flowers and by the action of the invertase enzyme present in the saliva of bees, *honey is* a natural product and has been part of our diet for millions of years, consumed by our ancestors, but only seasonally. In addition, it can be used as a replacement for sugar and sweeteners, with 20 to 30% higher power than sucrose to satisfy the sweet taste, which for most people is almost a necessity, it is superior due to its nutrient content. However, it should be noted that is contraindicated in children under two years of age because of the low acidity of their gastric juices, which can allow the development of the Clostridium botulinum germ from the spores that may be present in honey and may also be present in the soil and is the cause of infant *botulism*. Honey has only 22% water and a high content of 75% of various glucides, 35% fructose, 35% glucose,6% sucrose and less maltose and dextrins. It can contain up to 2% protein, has a low mineral content, and the vitamins present are of the B complex, plus C, D and E. Due to flavonoids and other phenolic compounds, it has antioxidant action, thus reducing free radicals. It strengthens the immune system with preventive action against cancer and infections.

The high glucid concentration determines osmolarity that produces the breakdown of bacterial membranes; thus it has antimicrobial and antiseptic properties. In this antimicrobial action, the content of the enzyme glucose oxidase also intervenes, which from oxygen produces hydrogen peroxide, which also dissolves the membranes due to its acidity. It prevents bacterial fungal and viral infections. Applied locally on wounds it prevents infection and facilitates healing, including burns.

For catarrh in the upper airways, it is a soothing pharyngeal cough remedy with superior action to dextromethorphan. When it is over a year old, due to poor storage (heat) a darkening could be observed due to the presence of hydroxymethylfurfural and glycation products, that can have carcinogenic properties.

Propolis

The product resulting from wax and saliva made by bees for the protection and defence of honeycombs, *propolis* is the subject of numerous scientific studies published in the last three decades with promising prospects for clinical application and various beneficial effects on health.[99,100] In addition to amino acids, lipid acids, vitamins and minerals, numerous bioactive phytochemical compounds from the group of polyphenols are already recognized. Some observations have been carried out on patients, but most of the studies have so far been carried out on experimental animals and cell lines using water or alcohol extract of propolis.[101,102] Propolis has an optimal action for the protection and development of the microbiota, inhibits pathogenic bacteria by suppressing adherence to cells and also increases the production by the microbiota of butyric acid, the main nutrient of the cells of the intestinal epithelium.[103]

The strong antioxidant, anti-inflammatory and antimicrobial action provide promising evidence for future clinical applications, particularly for neuronal and cardiovascular health. The antioxidant and anti-inflammatory action is also beneficial in chronic renal failure, with partial improvement in hypertension, creatinine, proteinuria and glomerulointerstitial damage.[104] Propolis extracts, due to their polyphenol content, including lycopene and turmeric, also showed benefits in experimental kidney injury in rats. Although propolis is considered non-toxic, allergic manifestations such as urticaria or dermatitis may occur, and a case of reversible acute renal failure has been reported with the suspension of the product.[105]

The great variation in bioavailability such as extracts in water or alcohol, local, seasonal and honeycomb variations and for different individuals according to absorption, which requires hydrolysis by intestinal enzymes and their particular microbiota, in addition to personal variations in renal excretion, still allow applications as a nutritional supplement aimed at prevention and adjuvant therapy of various diseases. Further experimental studies and careful clinical observations with pharmacodynamic and pharmacokinetic studies and the standardization of pharmaceutical preparations are necessary. For now, extracts in water or alcohol of propolis should be limited to local applications due to their optimal action for wound healing and oral health. Studies of plasma levels, renal and faecal excretion and clinical manifestations with the intravenous supply of one of the main active principles of propolis, pinocembrin, with doses of 20 to 150 mg, did not show any class of adverse effects.[106,107]

Many potentially beneficial health effects of propolis are inherent in its content of polyphenols, flavonoids and non-flavonoids, which are found in abundance in fruit and vegetables, where they will be considered in detail.

Proteins

Proteins, like lipids, are the most versatile substances in the body due to the multiple functions that they fulfil, as we can see in the following list that highlights only some of these functions.

- All enzymes are proteins acting as catalysts for the chemical reactions of metabolism, by facilitating and accelerating the chemical reactions that nutrients and their derivatives undergo in cell metabolism, either for growth, replacement or energy production.
- Some hormones such as insulin and glucagon are proteins and so are the tissue receptors for hormones for them to exert their action on.
- They fulfil defence functions through immunoglobulins and transport various hormones or an element as essential as oxygen, the latter through haemoglobin.
- There are also storage proteins such as lactalbumin and ferritin.
- They act as neurotransmitters and as an alternative source of energy.

They exert protective action against stress through heat shock proteins, with preventive action against neurodegenerative diseases.

Champerones, as packaging proteins, preserve the integrity of nuclear DNA against different toxins.

The basic structure of proteins is made up of long chains of amino acids coiled in a three-dimensional structure. This conformation begins to alter at 40°C and is lost at 60°C, a protein denaturation process with which they lose their action.

Essential amino acids

There are 20 amino acids in the body, of which eight cannot be synthesized and therefore must be provided by the diet, they are the absolute *essential amino acids.*[108,109] The eight absolute essential amino acids are isoleucine, valine, leucine, threonine, methionine, phenylalanine, tryptophan and lysine. As a memory resource, we can say:

iso va le thre me phe try ly.

Other amino acids, *arginine* and *histidine*, are optional as in certain circumstances, especially in childhood, the contribution from food is insufficient. Proteins of animal origin are those with the highest biological value as they are efficiently digested, absorbed and metabolized; they also contain all the essential amino acids. If we consider other protein sources such as cereals or pulses, it turns out that cereal proteins have lysine as a limiting amino acid and therefore must be supplemented with pulses, which in turn are deficient in the *sulfur amino acids* methionine and cysteine, that cereals have. In addition, in pulses, antinutrients such as phytates (insoluble chelates) with minerals reduce their absorption and also decrease the digestibility of proteins. By the main sources of protein of animal origin, we mean meat, offal and eggs and by meat, this includes beef, lamb, pork, poultry and fish.

Pork is medium-lean, as the fat is under the skin and not inside the meat. In poultry, commonly chicken or turkey, the leanest meat is found in breast meat.

Protein content in the aforementioned meat is around 14g%, but in small animals such as rabbits it is higher, up to 20g% and therefore the amount consumed should be less.

Among the absolute essential amino acids, a special reference to tryptophan is of interest.

Non-essential amino acids

In the metabolization of tryptophan, the neurotransmitter serotonin (5-hydroxytryptamine) is generated, a deficit of which creates memory, sleep, attention and appetite disorders, depression and even bipolar psychopathy.

Serotonin by mouth is not effective because it does not cross the blood-brain barrier. The prevention of these disorders is achieved by ensuring the presence of tryptophan in the diet, which is found in eggs, bananas, walnuts, almonds, chicken, turkey, chocolate and milk. Serotonin is referred to as the hormone of happiness or well-being, released from the central nervous system like *endorphins,* which are also referred to as well-being hormones due to the analgesic action released from the hypothalamus and pituitary glands. Serotonin is also released from the gastrointestinal tract. These hormones, serotonin and endorphins are also released by emotional states such as excitement, joy or orgasm.

Among non-essential amino acids, *glutamine* deserves special consideration; it makes up 60% of the amino acids of the muscle mass and neutralizes acids in the muscles avoiding cramps and states of acidosis. It is used by the kidney for ammonia synthesis, also in glutathione synthesis. Sources: parsley, spinach, nuts and meat. Glutamine can only come from raw vegetables however as it is destroyed by heating.

Water

Water is the fundamental substance, the *sine qua non* for life. Our body is 60% water in adult life, 70% in childhood and up to 80% in premature newborns. Almost all of the nutrients are dissolved in water, and it is the vehicle for them to reach the cells. Water is essential to maintain our temperature within narrow limits, between 36.8 and 37.2°C. even at times when there is great metabolic activity such as during exercise or in the postprandial period. In these circumstances, water acts as a coolant, preserving the structure and function of the proteins. This is due to the thermal property of water, its great latent heat during evaporation that allows it to absorb large amounts of thermal energy without raising its temperature too much and at the same time retain that energy by slowly releasing it.

Proteins are long chains of amino acids that are coiled in a three-dimensional structure.

At 60°C denaturation of proteins occurs due to alteration of their three-dimensional structure. Water is so fundamental to life, that it is not only present as an unavoidable component in all living beings, but our planet, among all the celestial bodies known up to now, has 70% of its surface covered with water, which in the oceans reach depths greater than those of its highest mountains and is at the same time surrounded by a blanket of clouds.

Water abundance on earth means extreme temperatures have been recorded, and these were in Libya 57.8ºC. and Wostok, in Antarctica -89.3ºC. At the same distance from the sun, our satellite, the moon has temperatures ranging from 123ºC to -153ºC and up to -247ºC in its craters.

Under current conditions, for a caloric intake of between 2000 and 3000 calories per day (30 to 40cal/kg) we lose approximately 2500ml of water (between 1000 and 1500 through skin and lungs, between 1000 and 1500 through urine and between 100 and 150 in faecal matter). Losses from the skin and lungs are mainly due to pulmonary evaporation and skin perspiration, both are insensitive losses and to a lesser extent due to sweating, which is a sensitive loss. These losses of 2500ml of water per day are replaced daily: 13% (more or less 300ml) by endogenous-produced water, by metabolizing nutrients, fats, proteins and glucides. The remaining 2200ml are provided by optimal meals that include, for instance: at least two or three servings of vegetables (90% water) six servings of fruit (80% water) two bowls of soup, 300g of meat, chicken or fish or two cups of tea or Yerba Mate, (which is a very *healthy* herb, *Ilex paraguariensis,* which has more antioxidants than green tea). Yerba Mate is originally from Paraguay and southern Brazil and is highly consumed in Chile, Argentina, Uruguay and Arab countries).

The water provided by these foods is rich in vitamins, minerals and enzymes. This means that we can consider the water in food as one more nutrient. Fresh vegetables, or those kept in the refrigerator for up to a week or in a freezer for months, maintain the integrity of their nutrients.

It is different if you consume, for instance: two cups of tea, Yerba Mate or coffee with milk with two slices of toast with butter or jam, a salad of lettuce and tomato, 100g of meat, one yoghurt, four buns and one piece of fruit; water provided from these foods will be about 900ml. You will therefore need 1500ml of complementary tap water. Flavoured soft drinks with sugar, sweeteners or high fructose corn syrup (HFCS) are in no way comparable to natural water for an optimal meal such as the aforementioned.

Water intake to increase caloric expenditure

After drinking 500ml of water for men or 375ml for women, it is observed in obese subjects that for 90 minutes *energy expenditure* triples. The effect of gastric volume and distension is ruled out because this is not observed after ingesting the same volume of water with isotonic saline content and the existence of osmoreceptors is postulated, probably by ionic channels. Part of the increase in caloric expenditure is also due to the action of the body to raise the temperature of the ingested water from 22 degrees if it is at room temperature, to 37 degrees (body temperature). Energy expenditure was recorded by 0_2 consumption and CO_2 production and occurred in men by the burning of lipids and in women, glucides.

An aqueous overload such as the one referred to, 30 minutes before meals, has also been shown to decrease caloric intake by 13%, but only in older subjects, between 60 and 80 years old and not in young people. The weight loss observed with this procedure for 12 weeks together with a hypocaloric diet was 44%, with 2kg of weight loss greater than with the hypocaloric diet alone.

Along with adequate nutrition and activity in programs to achieve weight gain and obesity corrections, the intake of water, preferably cold in the aforementioned modality, constitutes an easy-to-apply resource.[110,111]

Soft drinks and flavoured water

These drinks used as a contribution of water to the diet contain nothing but water, unnecessary calories and various additives which can create addiction. They are 'hollow water', without vitamins, enzymes or minerals and are types of water that cannot be qualified as nutritious. The labelling sometimes says that it contains minerals, but they are in such low concentration, as in all drinking water that they are inconsequential, and the labelling usually specifies water 'without sodium'. The sodium that any drinking water can contain, like other elements, is in such low concentration, labelled as trace, which is inconsequential. The advertising for sodium-free water is just as vicious as the advertising for cholesterol-free vegetable oils. In the advertisements for this type of drink, the recommendation to drink three litres per day is announced to meet the needs and preserve the hydration of the organism, without taking into account the endogenous water that originates from the metabolization of food and the water contained in food, which even in the case of a diet based largely on dense foods such as bread and pasta, provides 50% of our needs.

Subjects who get used to drinking excessive amounts of water that exceeds three litres per day consequently increase the volumes of urine with very low density. The kidneys can lose the ability to concentrate urine and they are exposed to dehydration if they decrease the volume of ingested water. On the other hand, in sports, excessive water consumption has been the cause of hyponatremia, that is, a decrease in the salt concentrations of body fluids. Normal subjects who do not have kidney disease do not need to control the amount of water to drink; this is naturally regulated by hunger and thirst.

Wine and other alcoholic beverages

With *wine*, as with many other things in life, wisdom is in the right measure. This especially deserves to be highlighted because it constitutes an emblematic example.

The content, mainly of *resveratrol*, *cyanidin*, *catechin* and *epicatechin*, are the determinants of the benefits referred to in the intake of wine. Its *antioxidant* action is beneficial for cardiovascular health, lowering LDL and platelet aggregation, and it has anti-inflammatory and anti-cancer activity. Resveratrol is found in the skin grape, and in red wine at a concentration of 15mg per litre, much more than in white wine. Alcohol favours the absorption of flavonoids but has a maximum dose that can be metabolized by the body without harmful effects. This means that wine, due to its beneficial properties for health, can be part of our usual diet, but always with moderate consumption. Excessive alcohol consumption has deleterious effects on health, deteriorating its nutritional status and affecting virtually all organs, mainly the brain, liver and pancreas. The daily dose of alcohol should not exceed 30g for men and 20g for women.

The alcohol contained in red wine is around 14% volume and since alcohol density is 0.794, it corresponds to 11g%, resulting in an allowable dose of 270ml (almost two glasses) per day for men and 180ml (a little more than one glass) for women.

White wine has lower alcohol content, around 11% volume, which corresponds to 8.7g%, resulting permissible dose of 350ml (a little more than two glasses) per day for men and 230ml (one glass and a half) for women, but due to its lower flavonoid content, it is not comparable to red wine.

The brain is one of the main areas that suffers from chronic alcohol abuse. However, the pathogenic mechanism has not yet been sufficiently clarified. Cognitive disorders and structural damage, cortical atrophy with loss of neurons occur in 50-75% of chronic alcoholism cases. Especially vulnerable is the frontal region of the brain, the limbic system and the cerebellum. Metabolic products of alcohol cause an increase in the generation of free radicals, which can lead to oxidative stress with cellular damage, especially in the brain, which has fewer antioxidants than other organs. In addition, dysfunction occurs in the folate metabolism which is involved in DNA synthesis. When DNA repair is not enough to balance its natural damage, genomic instability results in an increased risk for neurodegenerative disorder and *carcinogenesis.* This increases in subjects with the C667T mutation, common in the general population[1.12-114] the key enzyme methylenetetrahydrofolate reductase (MTHFR) in the folate metabolism. Due to the increase in the production of free radicals by reactive oxygen species and nitro oxidative stress and its high solubility, alcohol damages virtually all organs, especially, in addition to the brain, the liver, heart, pancreas, muscles, lungs and testicles. Mitochondrial DNA, lipid, and protein dysfunction with decreased adenosine triphosphate (ATP) generation lead to fatty liver disease, fibrosis, cirrhosis and carcinogenesis. Fatty liver in alcoholics and non-alcoholics causes increased lipids, cholesterol, obesity, insulin resistance and diabetes.[115]

Autophagy, a physiological process programmed in cellular homeostasis, creates an increase of by-products resulting from the metabolic oxidation of alcohol, which, through the enzyme alcohol dehydrogenase, generates acetaldehyde, a highly reactive product that is then transformed into acetate, (although less toxic), by the enzyme aldehyde dehydrogenase. The oxidation of alcohol occurs in the liver but also in the pancreas, the heart, the muscles and other organs, generating reactive oxygen species.

A mature brain is less affected than in the embryonic period by the protective action of the blood-brain barrier, but this is also altered by oxidative stress and by the release of intracellular calcium. Autophagy appears to play a major role in the production of pancreatitis, fatty liver, decreased brain weight and volume, loss of muscle mass and cardiac dysfunction, ventricular arrhythmia and sudden death. There are also alterations in the immune and endocrine functions, osteoporosis and damage to embryonic and foetal growth and development.[116]A decrease in vitamin absorption compromises the metabolization of nutrients, specifically, B_1 deficiency which is the cause of Wernicke Korsakoff syndrome.

Alcohol is not deposited in the body, it is eliminated through metabolization in the liver; the alcohol content in a glass of wine takes two hours to be eliminated, which interferes with the liver process for metabolization of food, lipids and amino acids and glucose. This leads to malnutrition with weight loss. Fatty liver and diabetes can be accompanied by weight gain and pancreatic calcifications can be observed.[117]

A substantial in vivo study in a controlled and randomized manner was carried out on the effects on the intestinal *bacterial flora* from the moderate intake of red wine. This study demonstrated the beneficial health effects of the probiotic and prebiotic action of polyphenols.

After ingestion for four months of 272ml daily of red wine, de-alcoholized red wine or 100ml of gin, inhibition in the development of pathogenic flora was verified, such as, to name just some of the best known, *Clostridium hystolyticum* and *Clostridium perfringens*, together with the increase in bacterial species with known beneficial actions for health such as bifidobacteria. This was observed as a consequence of the polyphenols and not of the alcohol. Parallel to the changes in the bacterial flora, there were metabolic changes determining reductions in the plasma values of uric acid, triglycerides, cholesterol and the LDL fraction of cholesterol, as well as decreases in blood pressure. Beneficial changes in the bacterial flora also mean actions favourable to intestinal health. The role of *Clostridium perfringens* in the initiation of inflammatory bowel disease processes and the progression of colon cancer is known. In addition, the stimulation in the development of a beneficial intestinal bacterin flora means the generation by fibre fermentation, of butyric acid, a fundamental nutrient of the intestinal epithelium with preventive action in colon cancer and ulcerative colitis.

The large intestine is the seat of an active fermentation process mainly of dietary fibre, carried out by the abundant flora of various bacterial species with up to 10^{12} cells per gram of faecal matter. Changes due to dietary factors and diseases lead to imbalances of the bacterial flora with consequent metabolic imbalances in the general economy with manifest repercussions on the state of health. In maintaining the bacterial balance in the intestinal lumen and consequently the metabolic balance in the general economy, the role played by polyphenols, phytochemicals present in especially red wine, as well as in tea, coffee, chocolate, fruit and vegetables is already unquestionable. Among these polyphenols is resveratrol, one of the most studied has confirmed its beneficial effects on intestinal health and the decreased risk of coronary heart disease. Seventy per cent of resveratrol is absorbed from the intestinal lumen. The beneficial effects on health have been observed not only in the prebiotic action but also in the reduction of systolic and diastolic blood pressure and the reduction of triglycerides, cholesterol and C-reactive protein. The decrease in these last two biomarkers has occurred in relation to the number of bacilli Bifidus present.[118,119] In *pasteurized* wines, probiotic properties are lost, and the addition of sulfites that are already naturally produced during fermentation inhibits malolactic fermentation.

Cow milk has lactase which is lost during pasteurising. This is why lactose intolerance occurs in adults. In addition, pasteurisation kills probiotics in milk as well as in wine. The pasteurization is carried out for infectological and commercial reasons for the conservation of the product.

Other alcoholic beverages with nutritional value due to their flavonoid content are hesperidin, limoncello and naliric and are referred to in Chapters 7 and 9.

Vitamins

Vitamins are essential substances, that is, the body does not synthesize them, except for vitamin D, therefore they must be provided by food. They are vital for life because they favour enzymatic reactions. In 1911 the first recognized substance of this type, thiamine, being an amine in its chemical nature, was called a vitamin. This substance was shown to be present in the husk of rice, with which the disease known as beriberi could be cured, hence it was called vitamin B, a substance that was shown to be water-soluble. Beriberi was epidemic in Asian countries that were fed refined rice, without the husk. Later, other diseases were discovered in which the responsible deficient substances were also called vitamins, assuming that they were also amines, although later it was seen that both vitamin C and the four lipid-soluble vitamins, A, D, K and E showed different chemical structures. All *water-soluble vitamins* are grouped into the B complex, numbering them successively after thiamine, which, because it was the first, was called B_1.

When ascorbic acid was discovered, although it is also water-soluble, due to its different actions, it is not integrated into the B complexes and is called vitamin C. When retinol was discovered, because it is lipid-soluble, having called the water-soluble ones 'B', it is called vitamin A. At present, 13 vitamins are recognized, nine are water-soluble and four are lipid-soluble. Vitamins act as cofactors of enzymes; they are co-enzymes, essential to facilitate metabolic reactions. Vegetables are an important source of vitamins, mainly water-soluble vitamins, B complexes and vitamin C, and among the lipid-soluble ones, from carotenes, vitamin A and to a lesser extent, vitamin K. With cooking the vegetables lose 30% of their content in water-soluble vitamins, and vitamin C is altered if the vegetables are left to soak for a long time, due to the action of the oxygen that the water contains.

Water-soluble vitamins

These are the *B complexes* and vitamin C.

The body does not have deposits of water-soluble vitamins; therefore their intake must be regular. An exception to this is vitamin B_{12}, which the body has deposits of that can last for years. In general, all the vitamins of the B complexes act in the metabolism of proteins, lipids and glucides and are antioxidants.

B_1, thiamine or antineuritic vitamin or antiberiberi

Its main action is in the metabolism of glucose for the release of energy, especially in the brain and peripheral nervous system. It acts in the transmission of the nerve impulse and the muscular and cardiac contraction. B_1 deficiency produces pictures of polyneuritis, with paresis, paralysis, tendon hyporeflexia, paralysis of the ocular muscles and memory disorders, loss of sensation, heart failure and alteration of the vascular walls with the production of oedema. B_1 deficiency usually occurs in alcoholic patients who may present with Korsakoff syndrome, brain damage and hallucinations. The term *beriberi* for B_1 deficiency disease in the Sinhalese language means "I can't"— or extreme weakness. It is present in meat, (liver and kidney), eggs, pork, fish and nuts. Fruit and vegetables contain it in small quantities, and abundant consumption of these foods ensures the necessary contributions.

B_2, riboflavin

This is involved in the metabolism of proteins, amino acids, lipids and glucides, particularly in cellular respiration. A deficit is usually associated with those of B_1 and B_3, producing eye irritation, inflammation of the cornea or keratitis, inflammation of the lips and mouth, cheilitis of the tongue, glossitis and seborrheic accumulation in the nasocutaneous folds.

Present in meat, offal, dark green vegetables and eggs, it is heat stable but sensitive to light.

B_3, niacin, nicotinic acid or vitamin PP, preventive of pellagra

It is part of two important co-factors of energy metabolism, nicotinamide adenine dinucleotide (NAD) and nicotinamide adenine dinucleotide phosphate (NADP) necessary to maintain the integrity of the skin, digestive mucosa and brain function.

B_3 deficiency produces the picture of *pellagra*, from the Italian for rough skin. The most affected skin is that of exposed areas, where it appears red, rough and scaly. There is inflammation of the digestive system from the mouth to the intestine manifesting with diarrhoea. Brain alterations give pictures of dementia with hallucinations, confusion and delirium. The clinical picture is referred to as the 4 ds: dermatitis, diarrhoea, dementia and death.

The picture occurs in cases of low protein intake with a diet sometimes based almost exclusively on corn.

Present in meat, chicken, fish and eggs.

B_5, pantothenic acid

It is part of acetyl-coenzyme A, which is involved in the formation of lipid acids, cholesterol and ketone bodies. An isolated deficiency is rare but can be seen in conjunction with riboflavin and thiamine deficiency and pellagra.

As its name indicates, it is widely distributed in food.

B_6, pyridoxine

It is involved in the synthesis of neurotransmitters, activates the transport of amino acids through cell membranes and the synthesis of docosahexaenoic and arachidonic acid from linoleic and linolenic lipid acids that regulate inflammatory processes and neurological functions. It is involved in the regulation of homocysteine levels, which when elevated increases the risk of heart disease. Pyridoxine deficiency as well as pantothenic acid and biotin are rare, except in the case of alcoholics. Seizures, dermatitis, anaemia, peripheral neuritis and skin and mucosal lesions similar to those referred to in B_3 deficits may occur. It is present in meat, chicken, fish, liver and some vegetables.

B_7/ B_8, biotin or vitamin H

It is a co-factor of several enzymes that catalyze reactions in gluconeogenesis, in the metabolism of lipid acids and amino acids. Biotin deficiency is rare, it can occur due to frequent ingestion of raw eggs since the avidin they contain is an antagonist of biotin. Biotin deficiency results in dermatitis, conjunctivitis, alopecia and abnormalities of the central nervous system. However, it is widely distributed in various foods.

B_9, folate

It is also often referred to as folic acid, but this is incorrect because folic acid does not exist in the body or nature. Folic acid or pteroylglutamic acid was synthesized by the Lederle laboratories in 1947, and in 1998 it was incorporated by the Food and Drug Administration in the United States as a supplement in wheat flour. Folic acid is transformed into folate in the liver, by the enzyme MTHFR, but a surplus of it, if not converted into folate, it has been argued, could have adverse effects. For this reason, at present the supply of folic acid has been limited for women as far as possible from one month before pregnancy and during pregnancy, reducing the doses after the first trimester. In this way, it decreases the incidence of neural tube closure defects, mainly myelomeningocele and anencephaly. Folate is involved in DNA synthesis and the conversion of homocysteine to methionine, reducing the concentration of homocysteine, a known risk marker for heart damage.

Vitamin B_{12}, cobalamin

Vitamin B_{12}, an extrinsic factor, is absorbed in the small intestine after binding in the stomach with intrinsic factors, secreted by the gastric mucosa. It is the last vitamin that was synthesized, in 1972. It has the most complex chemical structure and the only one that has a metallic element in its structure, cobalt. B_{12} has three synthetic variants. The most common has a cyano group, it is cyanocobalamin or B_{12a}, the others are hydroxocobalamin or B_{12b} and hydroxocobalamin or B_{12c}.

Cattle synthesize vitamin B_{12} by fermentation of the bacterial flora of the rumen and it is absorbed into their small intestine. Humans and rabbits can also synthesize it by the intestinal flora in the large intestine, but it is not absorbed since the absorption is done in the small intestine. In humans, a vitamin B_{12} requirement is met with minimal meat intake and the rabbit covers this deficit with coprophagia habits. It is essential in folate metabolism through methylation reactions to maintain intracellular folate levels. By interacting with folate, it lowers homocysteine levels, a known risk factor for heart damage, converting homocysteine into methionine. Also by interacting with folate, it intervenes in the synthesis and stabilization of DNA. Together with folate and methionine, it is involved in the production of red blood cells and hematopoiesis. It is of paramount importance for the maintenance of the functions of the central nervous system.

B_{12} deficiency occurs in pernicious anaemia due to congenital deficiency of production by the gastric mucosa of intrinsic factor, in patients who underwent gastrectomy, in infants exclusively breastfed by vegan mothers or in vegan subjects after several years of not eating food of animal origin who did not take supplements. The clinical manifestations are megaloblastic anaemia, irritability, anorexia, motor incoordination, ataxia, hyporeflexia, sensitivity disorders, paresthesias, glossitis and neuropsychiatric disorders to which growth retardation is added for children. The cobalamin requirements are very low, and the hepatic deposits last from three to six years but are covered exclusively with foods of animal origin. B_{12} deficiency implies a high risk of prematurity and low birth weight.[120]

Vitamin C or ascorbic acid, the anti-scab vitamin

Most mammals, except primates and guinea pigs, synthesize it from galactose and glucose. It is a lactone but the name of ascorbic acid is not related to its chemical structure, it derives from Latin and Greek and means 'without scurvy.' Indeed, it is the anti-scab vitamin. *Vitamin C* is essential for the formation of collagen or connective tissue since it is what unites everything and separates everything. Collagen is found in all organs between cells and is a structural component of the skin and mucous membranes.

Vitamin C is also an important antioxidant, which protects against free radicals, facilitates the absorption of iron in the intestine and reduces cholesterol. Supplements together with other antioxidants in patients with multiple cardiovascular risk factors show improvement in arterial elasticity and diameter and lipid and glucose metabolism.[121]Normal levels of vitamin C in plasma are between 0.8 and 0.9mg%, and severe deficiencies can give values even lower than 0.15mg%, with frank manifestations of the disease. The main signs are gum haemorrhages, petechiae, that is, pinpoint haemorrhages on the skin, oedema in the lower limbs, subperiosteal haemorrhages, that is, under the lining of the bones, muscle and joint pain and even brain haemorrhages.

In children, there are no gingival haemorrhages before teething, and somewhat similar to rickets, are observed due to bone demineralization with tracing of the bones in tracing lines, and, on both sides of the sternum the enlargement, (hypertrophy), due to the lack of calcification of the cartilage that join the ribs to the sternum. This configures the so-called costal rosary as in rickets, which differs from scurvy with painful palpation. It was Thomas Barlow who differentiated scurvy from rickets in children, which led to the designation of infantile scurvy with the eponymous Barlow's disease.

Hippocrates describes clinical pictures compatible with scurvy in 1500 BCE. Similar descriptions appear in the Egyptian Ebers Papyrus, but it did not appear in epidemic forms until the advent of the 15th century with the long overseas voyages, in which nutrition was maintained with the classic sea biscuit and other dry foods such as cereal grains, salted meat and seeds but no fresh food. At the time referred to as a sailors' disease, on prolonged voyages that could last 10 or more weeks it fatally decimated up to 80% of the crew.

In 1753, a Scottish surgeon of the British Navy, James Lind, noted that the disease was cured quickly with the ingestion of oranges or lemons. Vitamin C was isolated in 1927 and its chemical structure was specified by Haworth and Karrer, who shared the Nobel Prize for Chemistry in 1937, while in the same year the Hungarian Albert von Szent-Gyorgyi received the same award in Physiology and Medicine for his work on the biological functions of this vitamin.

The normal daily requirement of vitamin C is 90mg. in men and 75mg. in women. Under 60mg. daily the first signs of scurvy can appear. Grapes and cabbages have 90mg per 100g, oranges 50, lemons 40 and grapefruit only 30. With the intake of 300g of any of these fruits, more than the normal requirements are provided.

Smoking, due to the high oxidants content in tobacco smoke, requires higher doses. The need to increase to 3 or 5g of vitamin C has been reported for each pack of cigarettes a day. Smokers have low levels not only in their plasma but also in their leukocytes and various organs as well as in urine. Along with this, there is a decrease in defensive mechanisms against infections, a decrease in phagocytosis and immune responses, as well as an increase in capillary fragility and an increased risk of bladder cancer and poisoning by arsenic, lead and carbon monoxide. Without presenting the manifest clinical picture of scurvy, smokers show the biochemical picture that has been called smoker's scurvy. There has been abundant literature on all the harmful effects of smoking for a long time.[122-124] With regular meals based on natural foods of fruit and vegetables, such as that of our Paleolithic ancestors, approximately 390mg are ingested daily.

Linus Pauling, who was awarded the Nobel Prize in Chemistry in 1954 for his research on chemical bonds in the structure of complex substances and was a Nobel Peace Prize winner in 1962, recommended very high doses of up to 6 and 18g in 1972, of vitamin C to prevent colds. In 1979 he also argued for its beneficial anti-cancer effects. In 1986 he published a book *How to live longer and feel better* referring to the benefits on the risk of cardiovascular diseases along with vitamin E and their retarding effects on ageing, the 'anti-ageing' effect.

Given the authority of Linus Pauling, one of the most admirable scientific personalities, these postulates were widely disseminated, with the approval of the pharmacological industry due to the considerable increase in demands from the population. This story is relevant because it is still widely believed today in the population of the preventive action of vitamin C at high doses, 1g or more to prevent colds and 'flu. Later studies seriously questioned the benefits referred to, works that were objected to by Linus Pauling, who died at age 93 in 1994 whilst being treated for prostate cancer. In the course of his illness, he claimed that his habitual intake of high doses of vitamin C had delayed the onset of cancer for 20 years. Subsequent work could not demonstrate favourable effects on the prevention or evolution of colds, cancer or cardiovascular disease.[125,126] Only one publication from 2013 refers to a possible preventive effect of episodes of cold-induced asthma, which requires further studies in this regard.[127] Linus Puling was the initiator of orthomolecular "medicine" or the "right molecule"; the correct molecule. Something like natural substances beneficial to health, in high doses, that would have preventive effects for a disease.

Orthomolecular medicine would be like the other side of homoeopathy, which advocates that a substance that causes a disease, in infinitely small doses that in solution are impossible to quantify, leaves a molecular vibration and can cure the same disease.

Lipid-soluble vitamins

Lipid-soluble vitamins are the vitamins A, D, K and E. The body has deposits of these vitamins, mainly in the liver, so a daily intake is not essential.

Vitamin A, retinol or antixerophthalmic vitamin

Vitamin A has pleiotropic actions, that is, it has multiple effects. One of its active forms, retinoic acid regulates genes essential for cell growth and differentiation. It is involved from pregnancy in the development of the circulatory, respiratory, digestive, hemopoietic and immune functions. It is essential for the health of the epithelia in the skin and mucous membranes. It is of paramount importance through the formation of rhodopsin or visual purple in the retinal rods, to allow vision in dim light and night vision. Vitamin A deficiencies produce the ocular pathology called xerophthalmia, which causes photophobia, night blindness or nyctalopia, conjunctivitis, opacity and ulceration of the cornea that can lead to blindness, along with defects in tooth enamel, keratinization of the skin and mucous membranes, growth retardation and increased susceptibility to infections. It is found in animal products such as egg yolk, dairy, meat, liver, fish, vitamin A_1 from marine fish and A_2 from freshwater fish, poultry and cod liver oils. In products of plant origin, green leafy vegetables and orange or yellow fruit and vegetables, some carotenes, mainly beta carotenes, contain pro-vitamin A that the animal organism transforms into vitamin A that is deposited in the liver.

Vitamin D, cholecalciferol or antirachitic vitamin

Vitamin D acts on the metabolism of calcium and phosphorus, increasing intestinal absorption and reabsorption in the renal tubule.

By regulating plasma levels of calcium and phosphorus, it facilitates bone mineralization. It also appears to directly stimulate calcium entry into the bone by lowering intracellular pH. Evidence for anticancer action is being evaluated, especially for prostate, breast, intestine and lung and analogues with less hypercalcemic action.[128,129] Vitamin D has anti-inflammatory action and serum levels of it have been reported inversely related to autoimmune diseases and type1diabetes.[130-132] Vitamin D deficiency produces bone demineralization, *osteopenia* and to a greater degree, *osteoporosis*. This configures the picture of osteomalacia in adults, soft bones with an increased risk of fracture. In children, as a growing organism, *rickets* occurs with bone demineralization and the growth cartilage hypertrophies due to non-calcification. In infants, soft bones can be seen in the occipital area of the skull, craniotabes, a widening of the growth plates at the distal ends of the long bones and in the joints between rib and sternum. This configures the so-called costal rosary in childhood where the lower limbs are bent. Large and prolonged deficiencies of vitamin D in childhood produce acidosis, which aggravates the picture of rickets. The main source of vitamin D is synthesis in the skin by the action of ultraviolet sunlight.

D_3 or cholecalciferol from 7-dehydrocholesterol.

D_2 or ergocalciferol from ergosterol mainly from fungi.

Vitamin D is activated first in the liver and then in the kidney, by hydrogenation to form 1-25 dihydro cholecalciferol, which is the active or hormonal form of the vitamin. This is why vitamin D is a pro-hormone. Serum levels of vitamin D (25 OH D_3) should be between 40 and 70ng/ml. Low levels that are frequently found in up to 70% of the population, are alarming. Correction of this situation with bolus and daily or weekly supplementation protects against acute respiratory infection.[133] Low levels of vitamin D in up to 70% of the population can be mainly attributed to the following factors.

Little sun exposure by the population outside the summer period
Excessive use of sunscreen in the summer
High frequency of weight gain and obesity
Low egg consumption for fear of cholesterol

An increase in fat in the body has a sequestering effect on vitamin D due to its fat-soluble nature, which does not occur with the other fat-soluble vitamins, A and E present in various foods and K produced by the microbiota.[134].For this reason, people who are overweight or obese should receive a supplement of 1200 to 2000U per day.

In 1968, the American Health Association established a limit for ingestion of cholesterol of 300mg. per day and three eggs per week as a preventive measure for cardiovascular disease due to hypercholesterolemia. Since 1915 this is no longer valid; egg cholesterol is easily metabolized and no relationship has been seen between its intake and elevations of plasma cholesterol, so it is not justified to limit in our diet the great benefits of the important nutrients in eggs.

In experimental animals, it has been observed that phospholipids present in eggs inhibit the intestinal absorption of cholesterol.[135-140]

Vitamin K

This is also referred to as an anti-haemorrhagic vitamin. The name *vitamin K* comes from the German word *koagulation*. K_1 is the phytomenadione of plant origin, K_2 or menaquinone originated in the intestinal bacterial flora and K_3 or menadione is the synthetic vitamin K. It stimulates the hepatic synthesis of some of the factors necessary for blood clotting. These factors, called K-dependent, are factors II (prothrombin), VII, IX and X. Deficits can be observed in the newborn for which a vitamin K ampoule is given to prevent newborn bleeding. Also in intestinal malabsorption syndromes such as coeliac disease and pancreas fibrocystic disease, vitamin K deficiencies occur together with the other fat-soluble vitamins.

It is present in dark green leafy vegetables, fruit and meat. To a certain degree, it is also synthesized by intestinal bacterial flora.

Vitamin E, alpha-tocopherol or anti-sterile vitamin

Like vitamin C, *vitamin E* is a strong antioxidant agent. It protects the lipid structure of cell membranes, benefits the circulatory system and vision and reduces blood cholesterol levels. In rats, it has been shown to improve fertility and prevent miscarriages. Deficits can give hemolysis and neurological manifestations especially in premature babies and in malabsorption syndromes.

It is present in green leaves, broccoli, spinach, egg yolk, avocados, vegetable oils, dried fruit, almonds and walnuts.

Colophon

With the great advances in chemistry in the 20th century that allowed the identification, isolation and synthesis of the active principles in nutrients, specific supplements were recommended in high doses for natural nutrition in healthy states to prevent different conditions. Observational experiences up to now have been frustrating about the initial expectations or left questions about the possible adverse effects, as has already been proven with vitamins A and D. Each specific nutrient acts synergistically with the many other known and as yet unknown nutritional components present in natural foods. Diseases due to specific deficiencies of nutrients from food or metabolic origin require repairing contributions that are also specific to the present deficit as a therapeutic measure. For example, the therapeutic measures are the supply of vitamin D_3 for rickets or vitamin K_1 for hypoprombinemic haemorrhages. The advantages of natural foods for optimal nutrition under normal conditions are never surpassed by processed foods or supplements from the food or pharmaceutical industry.

Pedro Escudero, a great teacher of nutrition, in his book *Alimentación* (1934), in the part referring to vitamins, highlighted the essential need for natural foods.[141]

Minerals

Vegetables are an important source of *minerals,* both those that are found in greater amounts in the body, macrominerals and those that are found in small amounts, microminerals. Among the first we have:

Calcium

Cow's milk has a *calcium* bioavailability of between 30 and 35%, and almonds have a lower bioavailability, between 21 and 27%. Spinach is the vegetable with the highest calcium content, 210mg%, but its high content of oxalates means that it cannot be absorbed correctly. Therefore, those vegetables that have a low content of oxalates such as broccoli, Chinese kale, cabbage or kale should be selected.

Almonds and vegetables, being alkaline foods, determine the entry of calcium into the intracellular, promoting bone mineralization.

Magnesium

Magnesium integrates the chlorophyll molecule, which is the fundamental substance to take advantage of solar energy in photosynthesis. It is found in all vegetables in their green parts, generally the leaves, but in arid areas where there are vegetables, in order not to lose water, they reduce their foliage replacing the leaves with thorns; chlorophyll is in the stem, as we can well appreciate in cactus. Sources of magnesium include spinach, avocados and bananas.

In equilibrium with sodium, potassium and calcium, it regulates neuromuscular excitability and cardiac contractility. It is involved in the formation of neurotransmitters. With a calcium/magnesium ratio of 2:1, it avoids calcium precipitation, preventing lithiasis

Phosphorus

Phosphorus, in addition to participating together with calcium in bone mineralization, integrates important compounds that are energy stores. Compounds such as ATP, adenosine diphosphate (ADP), adenosine monophosphate (AMP) or creatine phosphate, act as energy batteries that by enzymatic reactions release energy for various functions such as chemical reactions of metabolism, muscle contraction or passage of minerals through cell membranes.

Phosphorus is also involved in compounds that regulate the concentration of hydrogen ions, that is, it maintains the acid-base balance of body fluids. These are the buffer compounds made up of a weak acid, phosphoric acid and salts of strong base, sodium and potassium phosphates. Compounds of sodium and potassium mono or diphosphate eliminate variable amounts of hydrogen ions in the urine, giving the titratable acidity of the urine, as another means of regulating the acid-base balance.

Sodium

Sodium along with chlorine, the two quantitatively most important chemical elements in extracellular fluids are the main determinants of extracellular volume. If the excess of these elements cannot be eliminated by the kidney, it leads to an increase in the volume of extracellular fluids, which can manifest as oedema. The lack of these elements leads to dehydration, which occurs when there is a significant loss, for example, due to diarrhoea.

Sodium bicarbonate in extracellular fluids regulates the acid-base balance.

Sodium in balance with potassium, calcium and magnesium regulates neuromuscular excitability.

Potassium

Potassium is the mincral quantitatively more important in cells. It intervenes as a co-factor of numerous enzymatic reactions. In thc extracellular, it regulates neuromuscular excitability together with sodium, calcium and magnesium.

Sodium and potassium, calcium and magnesium

Increasing the numerator or decreasing the denominator increases neuromuscular excitability. In particular, the preservation of normal potassium values in fluids is essential to maintain normal myocardial activity, avoiding electrocardiographic alterations that are exponential of rhythm disturbances and cardiac sufficiency. Likewise, hypotonia and hyporeflexia are observed in muscles in hypokalemia, while in hyperkalemia, perioral pallor is observed due to vasospasm.

The sodium/potassium ratio of 1:5 in the intake is particularly beneficial for cardiac function with preventive action on cardiovascular disease and arterial hypertension. A sodium/potassium ratio of 1:5 or even lower, close to 1:10 occurs with a diet based on natural foods: vegetables, meat and fruit, which naturally contain the requirements of these elements. The current Western diet with an abundance of processed foods and the addition of salt in its manufacture and during the ingestion and low consumption of vegetables and fruit leads to the sodium-potassium ratio being inverted and it can easily reach 5:1 and even more.

Chlorine

The importance of cations, Na + and K + (monovalent) and Ca ++ and Mg ++ (bivalent) has always been highlighted in the clinic due to their multiple functions, some of which we have referred to. *Chlorine,* on the other hand, has received much less attention, considering it almost a subsidiary element in the salts that provide sodium or potassium. However chlorine, in addition to regulating the volume of the extracellular fluid together with sodium, is also an important factor in the acid-base balance.

In the general population and from doctors in their therapeutic conduct, the risks of excessive sodium consumption have been widely disseminated, considering instead chlorine as a simple companion of various salts without health risks. However, chlorine, whether sodium chloride, potassium chloride or ammonium chloride, is acidifying and has various pathogenic effects that will be later referred to in relation to table salt, which is sodium chloride.

Among the microminerals we have:

Iron

Iron is primarily an integral part of haemoglobin for oxygen transport to all tissues.

For approximately the last 80 years, without a supplemental iron intake for infants, iron deficiency with consequent anaemia was common, which interferes with mental development. Among the causes of iron deficiency in childhood is the hidden loss of blood in faecal matter due to an inflammatory state of the intestinal mucosa in children fed with cow's milk, due to an immunological reaction to heterologous proteins (casein milk) other than those of breast milk (albuminous milk). To this is added not using iron pots in the kitchen and minor contact of the children with soil. Although iron is generously provided by vegetables, eggs, meat and blood sausage, breastfeeding should be the exclusive meal for infants during the first trimester.

In adult life, as causes of iron deficiency, we can refer to poor nutrition, gastrointestinal bleeding and metrorrhagia in women.

Iodine

Iodine is necessary for the production of thyroxin by the thyroid gland. The most active hormonal compounds are first, T_3 and then T_4, so named because they have three and four iodine molecules respectively. The thyroid, through the secretion of its hormones, regulates metabolism and consequently body weight and temperature. It also regulates immunity with antibacterial, antiviral, antiparasitic and anticancer action. It also regulates brain growth and development from the 15th week of gestation to three years and in women it regulates fertility. Elevations in cholesterol and alterations in respiratory and cardiac function also occur in hypothyroidism.

Iodine, iron and vitamin D deficiencies are among the most common in many regions.

Most iodine is in the oceans, which is why its deficiency is more frequent in areas far from the oceans. Iodine deficiency is also seen by ingestion of bromine or fluorine, toxic halogens, present in pesticides, insecticides, cosmetics, flours, water and oral hygiene products. Bromine is also present in soft drinks that contain brominated soya bean and corn vegetable oils as stabilizers and emulsifiers. Bromine and fluorine bind to iodine receptors, competing with them.

Sea fish and shellfish are important sources of iodine inputs.

Zinc

Zinc is necessary for the maintenance of immune function, collagen integrity, nail structure, cartilage, libido and sperm count, resistance to respiratory infections and wound healing. It is also necessary for the synthesis of insulin and nucleic acids, DNA and RNA and prevents macular degeneration. It is the only mineral whose content is scarce in vegetables; it is found especially in seafood, but also in edible mushrooms. The high calcium content in dairy products interferes with the absorption of iron and zinc.

Manganese, molybdenum, copper, selenium, chromium

Manganese acts as a co-factor of numerous enzymatic processes. It is involved in bone formation, growth and the integrity of skin surfaces. Manganese, like selenium and zinc, has an antioxidant action.

Molybdenum contributes to the metabolism and intestinal absorption of iron.

Copper together with iron is involved in hemopoiesis.

Selenium is necessary for antioxidant enzymes and is an element of glutathione peroxidase. It reduces the risk of cardiovascular disease and cancer and is important in the preservation of immune functions.

Chromium together with zinc and selenium are microelements necessary for metabolic functions, they are not abundant in vegetables, but a varied diet including mushrooms, seafood, meat, liver, chicken breast and eggs ensures the necessary requirements.

Table salt

Excessive consumption and its effects.

It should be taken into account that the excessive contribution of *salt*, which is sodium chloride, to the diet means an increase in the acid load that must be neutralized by the body. Sodium chloride is an acidifying salt. The usual diet of the vast majority of the population consists of processed foods based on cereals and pulses, whether they are grains or flours, forcibly subjected to cooking with added ingredients in various proportions of lipids, salt and sugar. Salt is also generously added to meat, salads, soups, tortillas, stews etc. at the time of preparation and even at the time of ingestion. Salt stimulates the appetite which leads to increased intake. This habit in the consumption of salt means that the ingestion of sodium chloride can reach 10g daily while international medical societies recommend that the ingestion of salt should be no more than 3g or even should be reduced to 2g per day. There is no doubt that the available scientific evidence shows us the deleterious effects on the health of excessive salt consumption, mainly due to the cardiovascular damage that it involves, high blood pressure and myocardial infarction. Also, the excessive consumption of salt causes deterioration of renal function and especially accelerates any existing decline due to previous diseases or due to the natural decrease in glomerular filtration rate with age.

Hypertensive patients, in addition to being medicated when necessary with hypotensive drugs, as the first therapeutic measure, are usually indicated for diuretics. Diuretic use in these cases is usually done for a long time, therefore potassium-sparing diuretics are preferred, or the diuretic indication is complemented with the daily supply of tablets or elixirs with potassium, gluconate or chloride salts. Prolonged diuretic medication is not without the risk of dehydration, especially in the summer and hyperkalaemia or hypokalaemia with paralysis and compromised cardiac function. Correcting the habit of adding salt to foods at the time of their intake is useful but not sufficient. The consumption of bread and pasta already means salt is being consumed.

For the common diet, we can say that, approximately, the natural salt content of foods represents 20% of the total intake, 25% is given by the salt added at the table or during cooking and the remaining 55% corresponds to the salt added during processing and manufacturing.[142,143]

An optimal meal should have a variety of vegetables and fruit daily, and occasional meat, including seafood. In addition to these foods from the vegetable and animal kingdom—forgotten by many— there is the third vital kingdom, fungi. Most of these foods, almost excluding meat, are eaten raw, without adding salt or sugar, but are seasoned with spices, such as turmeric, ginger, cinnamon and pepper. Some of the aforementioned foods, mainly meat and vegetables, are sometimes eaten after cooking in water. With this kind of meal, salt intake can be very low and depending on activity and time of year it can cause cramps. If this happens, the most recommended cure is to add a mixture of two parts of table salt and one of bicarbonate, which is more physiological in the proportion between sodium and chlorine. Likewise, after roasting meat without the addition of salt, it is preferable to common salt but added at the time of ingestion.

Cereals and pulses, that is flours and grains, such as pasta, bread and cakes are reserved for what we call occasional meals, on the occasion of a celebration, or sporadically for the simple reason of wanting to taste an old favourite dish.

Hyposodium salts

For about two decades now, the need to reduce salt consumption has been widely disseminated and more and more low sodium salts called ‘light’ or ‘diet’ are being offered on the market. *Hyposodium salts* have 60 or 70% less sodium, replacing sodium chloride with other salts such as potassium chloride or magnesium carbonate. These salts could be taken temporarily as a means of transition until modifying an eating behaviour where the most accepted foods are divided mainly into three categories: sweet, salty and tasteless.

Decreasing to the point of eliminating the addition of sugar and salt in our usual diet, our taste buds will gradually expand to encompass a wide and varied spectrum of flavours, some soft, subtle, others strong. We will gradually learn that grated raw carrots taste like carrots, as beetroot tastes like beetroot, and we will even discover that meat tastes like meat. The taste of each of these foods results from various combinations of the four basic tastes: sweet, sour, bitter and salty, to which is added the characteristic aroma of each of them. Some also accept the 5th taste, described in Japan in 1908 by R. Ikeda: *umami.*

Umami means tasty and it is a difficult taste to describe, it produces a velvety sensation on the tongue, induces salivation and enhances the flavour of many foods with a residual effect. The umami taste occurs in ripe tomatoes, soy sauce, breast milk, cow's and goats' milk, and in dashi foods from Japan, all foods that have significant glutamate content. The umami taste, the perception of which is referred to as localized, especially in the root of the tongue, is mainly due to glutamate and increases with the combination within narrow concentration ranges of salt and ribonucleotides (tosylate and guanylate). It is present for example when meat is combined with vegetables or in Italian cuisine, for example, Parmesan cheese with tomato sauce and mushrooms. The fact of enhancing the taste of some foods, especially canned meat, fish and vegetables, but not cereals, can be useful in the diet of the elderly, in whom, as a consequence of a decrease in the taste sensation, food intake may be decreased [144,145].

We can even reintroduce into the kitchen those flavours largely displaced by sugar and salt, the flavours of thyme, basil, rosemary, garlic, bay leaf, nutmeg and a pinch of chilli pepper. Pepper, in the not-so-young, even increases the feeling of well-being as it blocks pain receptors.

It should be noted that in the campaign to reduce salt consumption, the message that reaches the population the most is that this is based on the need to reduce sodium consumption, due to the damage that this implies to health, as well as how good potassium is.

As we have seen, some of the low sodium salts have sodium chloride replaced in part by potassium chloride and other salts. Both in the general population and among physicians there is almost total ignorance that the damage to health from excessive consumption of salt, and sodium chloride, is due not only to sodium but also to chlorine, as we detailed extensively in our book about body fluids.[146] The chlorine content in salt also participates in the high risk of arterial hypertension and independently of sodium it has other harmful effects on the health; the chlorides are acidifying salts. Sodium chloride is quantitatively the largest salt in extracellular fluid, including blood, followed by sodium bicarbonate. Chlorine and sodium make up 92% of the osmolarity (total dissolved particles), 53% corresponding to sodium and 47% to chlorine. In this way, not only sodium but also chlorine regulates the extracellular volume.

In addition to expanding the extracellular volume, an excess of sodium causes it to fixate on the arterial walls, which decreases the response to vasodilator agents in the body. A decreased response to vasodilators (decreased content) and an increase in extracellular volume (increased content) that occurs when the kidney is unable to eliminate salt excess, determines an increase in blood pressure. Normal blood pressure values should be less than 130/80, maximum/minimum, or systolic/diastolic; values that correspond to the height in millimetres of a mercury column. In the population, these values have been disseminated as 13/8 which corresponds to cm.

With so-called essential hypertension, it is worth saying that it is not due to kidney disease or another organic pathology. The suppression of salt in the kitchen and at the table and not incorporating processed foods into the usual diet is generally enough to achieve decreases in blood pressure by10 to 20 mm of mercury.

Other salts

Celery salt, sea salt, Himalayan salt

Other salts are not hyposodic. *Celery salt* is simply sodium chloride, common salt, flavoured with crushed celery seeds. The same goes for others, like garlic salt or onion salt. The taste and aroma of these salts can even lead to an increase in the addition of them to meals.

Another salt, used as an additive in gastronomy, especially in Chinese cuisine is monosodium *glutamate.* The Chinese restaurant syndrome, composed mainly of headaches, chest pain, numbness and burning in the mouth, a picture compatible with an allergic reaction, has been attributed, without having been conclusively proven, to the addition of this salt.

Sea salt, which originates from the evaporation of seawater, has 86% sodium chloride plus traces of other salts such as magnesium, manganese, potassium, calcium or iodine chloride. In the case of refined sea salt, the sodium chloride content is 99%.

Himalayan salt, from the mountains of Pakistan, is a rock crystal salt that has 98% sodium chloride and traces of other elements.

In both sea salt and Himalayan salt, the traces of the other salts mentioned are covered by a varied diet. With regard to iodine, the content is lower than that added to table salt to prevent goitre. Fluoride is also often added to table salt to prevent cavities. In addition to this, the difference with table salt is that the latter is subjected to more complex processing for refinement, including additives to avoid agglomeration, especially due to humidity.

Ethics

Living in balance with the natural and social environment is a must.

Not doing harm but producing or promoting good through the constructive development of oneself and others and preserving the environment is the essence of the ethical development that we must achieve.

Currently, there is a great wealth of valuable knowledge both on adverse factors for health and other benefits for it.

There is no doubt about the deleterious effect of smoking mainly on the respiratory system and not only in relation to lung cancer but also to chronic obstructive pulmonary disease.

There is also no doubt that the conjunction of a sedentary lifestyle and overeating are conditions of serious metabolic imbalances. Both situations cause not only high mortality but also a tremendous deterioration in the quality of life with serious limitations until reaching terminal states. This transcends the individual projecting into high economic and social costs. They are also the cause of family disturbances and suffering.

Likewise, there are no doubts about the health benefits of a regular diet based on a predominance of various vegetables and fruit complemented with meat and certain spices, which beyond their value as seasonings have various actions to optimize metabolic functions, which allows them to be considered as functional foods. To this must be added a moderate practice of exercise, preferably outdoors with regular sun exposure. With this, all kinds of deficiencies are avoided, health is preserved, diseases are prevented and ageing is delayed, which as a physiological process, will allow a long and full life.

We live in a complex, multifaceted society, with great technological development, far removed from what we could say is a pastoral life.

Large business organizations, mostly multinationals, present skillful journalistic campaigns not only for household appliances, cars, mobile phones, cosmetics and toothpaste, but also for processed foods and beverages. The packaging of biscuits, cereals, powders or beverages listed as energizers or nutritional supplements are permanently renewed.

Companies that produce beverages, processed foods and nutritional supplements allocate significant financial resources to promote the consumption of these products, attending marketing seminars to ensure maximum profitability and not the maximum benefit for health.

Faced with this permanently active and always-renewing advertising campaigns, there is an absent or almost absent state-funded program for nutrition and food education.

Vegetables, fruit, meat and mushrooms

We said vegetables, fruit and meat are all essential foods because they metaphorically promote 'biological virtues' for our body.

Vegetables

Taking into account their botanical characteristics, we say that *vegetables* are the edible parts of a plant that are neither the fruit nor the seeds.

Tomatoes, squash, courgettes and cucumbers are *fruits* and cauliflower, broccoli and artichokes are flowers or a set of flowers, or inflorescences, but are generally considered vegetables. In addition, the best-known fruit, such as citrus fruit, watermelons, melons, plums, pears, grapes, pomegranates, apples, bananas and many others, have a nutritional composition similar to vegetables.

Vegetables and fruit contain mainly complex glucides and a large amount of water, fibre, vitamins, and minerals and have a lower protein and lipid content, except for avocados, coconuts and dried fruit, which with lower water content have high-quality lipids; omega-3 lipid acids.

It is also important to note that vegetables and fruit contain innumerable phytochemicals, mainly more than 10,000 *polyphenols,* many of which have beneficial effects to preserve health and assist in the treatment of numerous diseases, among other actions, as antioxidants, anti-inflammatories and anti-cancer, which will be discussed later.

Vegetables and fruit leave alkaline residues when metabolizing, which maintains the acid-base balance, neutralizing the residual acid load when metabolizing foods from the animal kingdom.

Without a regular and sufficient intake of vegetables and fruit, a diet based on a daily or almost a daily consumption of meat, (be it beef or lamb, pork, poultry, fish or shellfish, to refer only to the most frequently consumed), adding to this cereal, pulses and dairy products, cheeses and yoghurts, and the strong acid load that this implies produce physiological responses that over the years significantly increases the risk of a deterioration in health.

Vegetables and fruit, due to their high water content, between 85 and 95% and their low lipid content, between 0.2 and 0.24g% make a low caloric intake, between 12 and 25kcal/100g derived mainly from glucides, between 0.9 and 2.7g% and proteins, between 0.9 and 1.8g%.

The best salts for our body are those found in vegetables, meat and fruit that provide us with sodium, potassium, calcium, magnesium, chlorine, phosphorus, iron, manganese, cobalt and a few others. Only zinc is scarce in vegetables and red meat or poultry but is found especially in seafood and mushrooms.

In addition to these common properties of fruit and vegetables, those vegetables and fruit with special characteristics that deserve to be highlighted are worth considering.

Cooking vegetables by boiling or blanching leads to a significant loss of minerals and glucides but is largely avoided by steaming them or using a pressure cooker.

The aforementioned is especially useful for cooking chard and spinach if they are consumed frequently and in abundance, since nitrosamines, substances with a possible carcinogenic effect, are also inactivated, which are generated from nitrates that may be present in these vegetables in excessive quantity.

Also steaming in a pressure cooker is convenient for cabbages, such as cauliflower or broccoli, which contain thiocyanates that act as antinutrients by reducing iodine absorption.

Due to the thermolability of enzymes, vitamins and other micronutrients such as flavonoids, which act synergistically as antioxidants avoiding cell damage from free radicals, a large part of vegetables must be consumed raw.

Vegetables can be kept for a week in a refrigerator at 8ºC, or in a freezer for up to 15 days in plastic bags with holes, in this way they retain all their properties

Vegetables such as lettuce, spinach, arugula, endive, chicory, celery, radishes, basil or parsley, chopped in 1cm pieces, along with grated carrot, beetroot or pumpkin can be mixed with fruit cut into cubes and covered with whole lemons and oranges with the peel grated and previously frozen. In this way lemons and oranges have more nutritional value and lemon is less sour and favours the preservation of the vegetables, which in any case, if the vegetables are cut as we suggest, should be done immediately before consumption.

This makes vegetables together with fruit, that is foods from the vegetable kingdom, indispensable and irreplaceable for the promotion and preservation of health, foods that must be indispensable complemented with those from the animal kingdom and subsidiarily fungal.

Polyphenols interact with *nitric oxide* preventing hypertension and atherosclerosis, protecting cell membranes from lipoperoxidation, protecting against macular degeneration and improving immune status. They modulate the production of collagen, which favours the preservation of the skin's structure, as well as a photo-protective effect with anti-UV action.

The brain has fewer antioxidants than other organs and is thus more susceptible to neuronal damage due to oxidative stress, an important factor involved in the increase in neurodegenerative diseases in elderly patients. The anatomical location and the blood-brain barrier are important means for central nervous system protection against various injuries, but they constitute a disadvantage for some agents that experimentally show a neuroprotective effect to having access to neuronal tissue.[147]

Polyphenols decrease the generation of free radicals. They have a neuroprotective action and optimize neuronal function, not only as antioxidants but also to reduce inflammatory stress, preventing the progression of neurodegenerative diseases.[148]

Fruit and vegetable polyphenols have been observed to cross the blood-brain barrier, specifically caffeic acid, and modern methods are being explored that increase the bioavailability of polyphenols in general through nano-transporters for the treatment of neurodegenerative diseases.[149-151] There are promising prospects for the use of *pinocembrin* in Alzheimer's disease, due to its protective action against beta-amyloid toxicity by inhibiting receptors for advanced glycation products and through regulation of mitochondrial apoptosis.[152]

Leaves, stems, tubers

Leaves: *lettuce*, chard, spinach, chicory, endive, radish, parsley, watercress, celery, beetroot and leeks that are used without separating the stems from their small bulb, can be used to make an omelette.

Vegetable leaves, especially chard and spinach, are a source of *nitrates*, a recognized bioactive phytochemical with the cardioprotective property through its conversion into nitrites in vascular endothelium and is present in saliva. Its beneficial actions for cardiovascular health translate into a decrease in blood pressure, optimization of endothelial function and platelet aggregation and reperfusion in areas of ischemia due to atheroma plaques. However, excess nitrates and nitrites can produce methaemoglobinaemia, which occurs mainly with water from wells and also tobacco smoke. In meat and sausages with preservatives, nitrates and nitrites in the digestive system with protein amines produce carcinogenic nitrosamines.

In greenhouse vegetables grown with little sun, the plant does not use all the nitrate for proteins and with the use of nitrate fertilizers, this increases in the leaves. For this reason, chard and spinach should be given in moderation until one year of age. The WHO considers it prudent not to ingest more than 500 g. of chard in order not to exceed the intake of nitrates.[153,154]

Stems: asparagus, leek, green onions.

Tubers: they constitute the thickened part, underground, that some stems have: beetroot, carrots, sweet potatoes, radishes and green onions.

Potatoes are not included because we do not recommend them for usual meals due to their solanine content; an alkaloid, a natural pesticide, which increases when germination begins, which is why many potatoes come dirty and covered with charcoal as this inhibits their germination. The toxicity increases if it is cooked with the peel. It can cause diarrhoea, vomiting, hallucinations and a drop in blood pressure. For a usual diet, the potato can be replaced by sweet potato, with the advantages of its lack of toxicity and its pleasant taste, or fried sweet potatoes if preferred. After eating fried foods with the reuse of vegetable oils, endothelial damage occurs, and arterial dilation of 7% drops to 0%.[1]

Studies continue on the effect of various nutrients on cardiovascular risk induced by endothelial dysfunction, oxidative stress and postprandial inflammation, as well as on the favourable effects mainly of polyphenols contained in fruit and vegetables.[156,157] The endothelial function requires optimal omega-6/omega-3 avoiding glycation due to excess sugar.

It has been reported that trans lipids and megatrans oxidation products of vegetable oils interfere with the capacity of endothelial cells to generate nitric oxide, a determinant of arterial dilation, which implies a risk of cardiovascular damage and erectile dysfunction, even interfering with the action of products such as Viagra[158.]

Beetroot

Among the tubers, the numerous properties that are particularly beneficial for health are little known, both in fermented *beetroot* to preserve the microbiota, and in the form of a smoothie due to its content of vitamins, minerals and phytochemicals with anti-inflammatory and antioxidant actions. It is also worth highlighting its content of inorganic nitrates that the body transforms into nitric oxide, a vasodilator that increases the supply of oxygen to cells and the efficiency of mitochondrial metabolism. All this does make beetroot juice considered a functional food, metaphorically referred to as the 'blood of the earth' and is discussed in more detail with bibliographical references in Chapter 7.

Bulbs

They are tubers surrounded by leaves: onion and garlic. The leaves may surround the tuber in layers, tunicate or cataphiles.

Some vegetables have edible tubers and leaves, such as beetroot or both the stems and the leaves, such as celery and chicory, or both the bulb and stems such as green onions and leeks.

Broccoli

Broccoli contains glucoraphanin, which is converted into *sulforaphane* by the action of the myrosinase enzyme. The enzyme is sensitive to heat, but sulforaphane is not. It has been reported that sulforaphane ingested three times a week can promote the dissolution of atheroma plaques. How to prepare it to achieve this action is described in the final chapter.

Broccoli and to a lesser extent *cauliflower* have been reported to be associated with a lower risk of myocardial infarction, cancer development, neurodegenerative diseases and atherosclerosis, but the evidence in humans is limited. It also increases the level of testosterone which protects muscle and joint tissue.[159]

Pesticides, herbicides, plastic containers, cosmetics and environmental contamination by petrochemical products, act as *xenoestrogens* that cause an increase in abdominal fat. This is neutralized by crucifers, such as broccoli, cauliflower, cabbage or Brussel sprouts.

Watercress

Watercress is a very important source of nutrients. Taking into account the content of vitamin A, D, K, E, B_1, B_2, B_3, B_6, B_9 and C, of the minerals potassium, calcium, iron, zinc, fibre and protein, in a study of the nutritional density of fruit and vegetables it was placed with the maximum score of 100.

Parsley

Parsley is mentioned as this vegetable is not currently used as much as it was two or three generations ago when it was almost a daily component of the diet in many different meals. The high content of calcium, and iron, in addition to magnesium and potassium is remarkable. In vitamins, those of the B complex stand out, especially B_2, riboflavin and B_9, folate, as well as vitamin K and beta carotenes. Its high folate content reduces the level of homocysteine, a risk marker for cardiovascular disease.

In vitro and in vivo studies in animal and human samples show its high health-promoting properties, with numerous active principles, and high phenolic contents that are strongly antioxidant, prevent oxidative stress and consequent diseases, protecting the DNA and mitochondria. Its proven antiproliferative effect in colon cancer implies potential clinical applications.

The active ingredient, flavonoid glycosides of quercetin, luteolin and myristicin have antitumour properties, reducing the effect of *carcinogenesis*-inducing free radicals.[160]

It should always be consumed fresh to avoid oxidation in salads and pasta, stews, soups and infusions. For tea with ginger and cinnamon, see the recipe in the final chapter; it is recommended as a digestive as it prevents gastric acidity and favours glycemic control.

Vegetable sprouts, mainly soya beans and alfalfa are readily available, have a higher content of nutrients, minerals, lipid acids, protein and fibre than the adult plant and can be regular ingredients in salads.

Garlic

Since ancient times, *garlic* has been attributed beneficial health properties such as antioxidant, anti-inflammatory, antimicrobial, antitumour, glycemic regulation and a reduction in the risk of cardiovascular disease, however, controlled studies are lacking to confirm such effects.[161,162] Studies carried out with allithiamine, one of the compounds in garlic, suggest that the significant suppression of pro-inflammatory changes produced by advanced glycation end products (AGEs) induced by hyperglycemia, with consequent endothelial dysfunction, are due to its powerful antioxidant and anti-inflammatory action.[163.]

Vegetables and fruit, except for dried fruit such as nuts, almonds and hazelnuts and others also rich in lipids such as avocados and coconuts, have high water content, 80 to 90% of which the glycemic load and consequent caloric intake are low. Likewise, and due to the high fibre content, which slows down the absorption of glucides, the glycemic index is low, generally between 35 and 46, somewhat higher between 38 and 46 for kiwi, banana and pineapple and only cherries reach 72.

Fruit

Apple

An *apple* of 195g has 22.3g of glucides, 0.7g of proteins and 0.8g of lipids. Among the glucides, 9.5g corresponds to fructose, that as will be seen when treating the subject of Maillard reaction, or glycation, is highly reactive, even more than glucose, but due to its high fibre content, the glycemic index is low, at only 38. However, the consumption of fructose should be limited, which corresponds to 400 or 500g of fruit, with two apples, of approximately 200g each we already have almost 50% of the recommended intake of fruit.

This results in the saying with which we started this book: "An apple a day, keeps the doctor away", an apple or maybe two, is the prudential measure as regards apple intake, thus leaving room for another 200 or 300g of other fruit, for variety in taste and the complementation of other components that are not in apples. We already mentioned the antioxidant, antiallergic and anticancer action of the apple, derived from the flavonoids it contains, from *quercetin* which is especially concentrated in the peel. Like all flavonoids quercetin is heat-sensitive, it is inactivated by heat, which is why the apple should be ingested as we said, fresh, with the skin on and not baked.

The ursolic and oleanolic acid isomers, also present in apple peel and pears, blueberries and cherries, also have anticancer properties[164] and are being studied in pharmaceutical preparations that improve bioavailability for therapeutic purposes.[165] The stimulating effect on muscle mass and fat burning has also been proven in experimental animals. Chewing an apple with peel can be somewhat difficult, this can be avoided with a grated apple ingested in a salad or a cold or warm infusion. In any case, the heart should be discarded, with two or three seeds contained per unit.

Apple seeds contain toxic cyanide that in a small amount does not imply any risk. The seeds that are unintentionally ingested are eliminated without being digested. Cyanide is released only if the seeds are chewed, which produces a toxic action, and in a number greater than 10 or 15, (fewer for a child).

Citrus

Mainly oranges, tangerines, lemons and grapefruit, plus limes and bergamot.

Citrus fruit can be considered the most important fruit for health since, being among those with the highest availability and consequently the highest consumption; they are exceptionally rich in phytochemicals.

Oranges

Oranges, in particular, have been the subject of numerous studies, and have the highest antioxidant content of all fruit, with 170 phytochemicals, polyphenols and among them, 60 flavonoids. They also contain glutathione, with antioxidant, anti-inflammatory, anti-tumour, anti-allergenic, anti-viral and anti-proliferative action. In the peel, the coumarin is anti-cancer. They are also rich in anthocyanins and lycopene, (especially red oranges), carotenes (precursors of vitamin A) (retinol) and folate.[166,167] They exert preventive action against cardiovascular disease, diabetes, cataracts, arthritis, intestinal inflammation and Alzheimer's disease. The well-recognized richness of vitamin C, typical of all citrus fruit, increases the bioavailability of iron by stimulating its absorption, which is especially important in women of childbearing age, vegetarians and athletes.

Bananas

Carotenoids, polyphenols and phytosterols are important components with a strong antioxidant action of proven benefit to preserve heart health, to which is added very low sodium and high potassium content.

Bananas are among the vegetables with the highest antioxidant capacity, as are broccoli, sweet potatoes and ginseng.[168]

The high fibre content gives the banana eupeptic properties.

Its easy digestibility makes it suitable for coeliac disease sufferers.

Carotenoids protect against LDL oxidation, LDL and glucose decrease. In prediabetics and diabetics, it can reduce cardiovascular risk.[169,170]

In acute diarrhoea, they are indicated for their easy digestibility, especially cooked in the oven until the skin turns black and the pulp yellow.

Papaya

Native to pre-Columbian America, cultivated by the original peoples in the tropical zone, currently its cultivation extends to the subtropical zone, including Asia and Africa.

The content of vitamin A, C, B_1, B_2, B_3 and B_9 is remarkable; also the minerals calcium, magnesium, phosphorus, iron, sulfur, silicon and potassium; it is also abundant source of fibre. The alkaloid papain in its peel stimulates digestion and protein assimilation.[171,172] It is digestive eupeptic, anti-inflammatory, intestinal antiparasitic and favours healing. Until 30 or 40 years ago there were pharmaceutical products such as Anatase and Papasine and at the end of the 1960s in the United States an injectable was promoted with: "Carica *papaya* injected into the buttock" as a fast and very effective anti-inflammatory and consequently musculoskeletal analgesic, today fulfilled less effectively by NSAIDs such as ibuprofen or paracetamol.

Paraphrasing that anonymous Anglo-Saxon saying with which we began this book: "an apple a day keeps the doctor away", in some regions of Ibero-America it is said: "a papaya a day keeps the doctor away".

Mango

Mango is also cultivated in tropical and subtropical areas. The content of vitamin C is higher than that of lemons, it also contains vitamin A carotenes that preserve eye health. The high content of polyphenols and fibre gives it glutathione antioxidant properties, which reduces the risk of chronic diseases and cancer. It also has anti-inflammatory, hypotensive and antimicrobial action against bacteria, viruses and fungi.[173,174]

Avocado

Avocado should be a frequent nutrient in our meals mainly due to its high content of good quality lipids, it is rich in omega-3 lipid acids precursors through a hepatic synthesis of docosahexaenoic acid that in adults and especially in senescence could favour the preservation of cognitive development and memory and could have preventive action on Alzheimer's disease.

Lipids, abundant in brain tissue, act as neurotransmitters allowing an inter-neuronal connection. The abundant content of phytochemicals such as polyphenols has antioxidant power, and the content of carotenoids and vitamin E is also important. Studies with cell lines, with animals and in the clinic show benefits in chronic cardiovascular and osteoarticular diseases. In addition to the already demonstrated health benefits derived from the pulp, there are also observations of possible anticancer actions that could be derived from the consumption of the seeds, but scientific evidence is still lacking in this regard.[175-177]

Pomegranate

Due to its tannin, anthocyanin and lycopene content, it has antioxidant, antiatherogenic, and antihypertensive action, inhibits LDL oxidation and decreases the risk of heart attack

Pomegranate juice administered for one year in patients with coronary artery stenosis showed a 30% reduction in stenosis compared to a 9% increase in controls.[178]

Tomatoes

Tomatoes, like all fruit and vegetables, for the full use of their components, must be eaten fresh, since with cooking various amounts of vitamins and minerals are lost and flavonoids are inactivated. However, fried tomatoes, or in the preparation of sauces, increases the bioavailability, with its health effects, of the abundant *lycopene* they contain, which, unlike *flavonoids*, are thermostable.

Common tomatoes used in salads contain lycopene at 3mg/100g and this is ten times higher in small tomatoes. The highest content occurs in tomatoes that ripen on the plant outdoors in the summer. Oils facilitate their absorption and, unlike most plant compounds, they are released especially when cooking. For this reason, it is advisable to eat not only fresh tomatoes but also tomatoes that are fried or in tomato sauce. In this way, the activity of lectins and allergenic antigens is also mitigated in susceptible subjects.[179]

Lycopene is a lipid-soluble colourant and is abundant in all red fruit and tubers, especially tomatoes, red grapefruit, watermelons and apricots. Lycopene, like the better-known beta carotene, is part of the family of carotenoids, compounds not formed in our body, but obtained through food, synthesized by plants and microorganisms.

The interest aroused by lycopene in recent years is due to several epidemiological studies that suggest that high consumption of them determines a lower risk of myocardial infarction and cancer, especially of the prostate. Likewise, a high antioxidant capacity has been observed, which defends our body from the damage of an excess of free radicals.[180]

Resveratrol and lycopene have been specially studied for their protective effect on the skin, preventing premature ageing with hyperpigmented spots and wrinkles and injuries caused by the oxidative action of ultraviolet rays during sun exposure.[181]

Cocoa

Cocoa and coconut are two fruits that deserve special consideration for the lipids they contain. In both, the lipids, despite being of vegetable origin, are not liquid in their natural state but solid, so it is not appropriate to call them oils, but cocoa butter and coconut butter.

Cocoa is a fruit of about 20cm in size that has a whitish paste inside where the seeds are. The cocoa mass must be distinguished from the cocoa powder, which is the solid, ground part, which also contains 25% cocoa mass, which also has theobromine similar to caffeine.

Chocolate is a mixture of cocoa butter and sugar with or without milk; the percentage of cocoa it contains determines its flavonoid content. In dark chocolate with 65% or more cocoa, 45g has 54mg of flavonoids, in milk chocolate with 25% cocoa, the same amount gives 13mg and white, which according to the Argentine Food Code should contain no less than 25% cocoa, has 0 flavonoids. All have slightly more than 500% calories, the bitter black with less than 46% sugar and the semi-bitter between 46 and 55% sugar.[18] The consumption of 63g of dark bitter chocolate per week lowers LDL and increases HDL· percentages and reduces the risk of brain haemorrhage but controlled studies are lacking to confirm such effects.

Coconut

Coconut contains 91% saturated lipids, 6% monounsaturated and 2% polyunsaturated. They do not become fat deposits as they are fast sources of energy, and, unlike olive oil, are resistant to oxidation. The saturated fatty acids are short and medium-chain; 52% is given by lauric acid, of an intermediate chain of 12 carbons, 19% by myristic acid of 14 carbons and 10% by palmitic acid, of 16 carbons. Other saturated fatty acids are caprylic 9% of 8 carbons and decanoic 10% of 10 carbons. Among the monounsaturated fatty acids, there is oleic 8%. Lauric acid stimulates immune processes and is antibacterial. A study carried out on women with an increase in abdominal circumference greater than 88cm (abdominal obesity) with supplementation of 30ml of coconut butter or soya oil for 12 weeks seemed to show a reduction in abdominal circumference with coconut butter, together with an improvement in the cholesterol lipid in its HDL and LDL fraction.[183, 184]

Another study on experimental animals showed that in allergies induced by sensitization to ovalbumin, the coconut butter supplement reversed the inflammatory process and bronchial hyperresponsiveness by controlling oxidative stress by interaction with nitric oxide.[184]

Kiwi fruit

Kiwi fruit is particularly rich in vitamin C. One unit has 117% of the daily requirement of this vitamin. It is also worth noting its content of vitamins E and K along with a high content of fibre and antioxidant activity.

Berries

They are small, strongly coloured red and dark blue bush fruits, such as blueberries, blackberries, strawberries, raspberries and currants. They are especially rich in antioxidant flavonoids, including resveratrol, also in vitamin C, calcium and potassium. *Berries* can be frozen.

From the blueberry extract, there are pharmaceutical products such as IU 400, IU 600 and Blue King, which have proven preventive action against urinary infection by preventing bacterial adherence to the epithelium.

Figs and prickly pears

Figs and *prickly pears* are very appetizing fruit with healthy nutrient content of fibre, calcium, magnesium, potassium and glucides with a low glycemic index. As fresh fruit they can be part of our usual meals; not due to medical limitations but because they are of short seasonal production, (except for dried figs, but this is due to the loss of water, although they have triple the concentration of nutrients, also triple their caloric value, should be eaten no more than 4 or 5 units). As summer fruit, the opportunity for consumption should not be missed due to the delight of their flavour and rich content of natural glucides that give satiety by reducing caloric consumption. Figs are also attributed to preventive action for macular degeneration, a common pathology in people over 60 years old[185] and should be eaten in their natural state and chewed, which begins their digestion due to the action of ptyalin, an enzyme present in saliva.

Some fruit, such as grapes, plums, peaches, apples and medlars, should preferably be eaten with their peel on.

Lemons and oranges that have not been fumigated with insecticides or fungicides can be placed in the freezer and then grated to facilitate their whole consumption, for the complete use not only of their fibre but also of antioxidants. The grated peel can be added in infusions at a temperature below 60° to avoid the inactivation of antioxidants and it can also be added to fish and salads.

The consumption of fruit and vegetables, by habit, is done separately but there is no reason why this should be practised systematically. At breakfast, for example, you can mix chopped fruit with vegetables like lettuce, including tomato sauce, to take advantage of lycopene.

Also as a possible alternative, especially in the summer, the classic fruit smoothie with ice is much better if it is made by combining fruit and vegetables.

Dried fruit

Nuts are walnuts, almonds and *hazelnuts*, chestnuts and pistachios. All are high in healthy lipids; omega-3. Regarding the aforementioned aspect of the importance of the nutritional contribution of lipids for brain function, the similarity in the appearance of *walnuts* with the cerebral hemispheres is at least curious. Such similarity could be considered a paradigm of that anecdotal theory of signs that announces other similarities, naturally due to chance, such as the shape of the apple that mimics the heart, or the tomato homologated with the prostate on which it exerts favourable effects due to its lycopene content. Although we cannot validate the theory of the signs, it is useful as a memory aid to remember the nutritional benefits of walnuts.

In *almonds,* the high protein content stands out, and therefore, by adding glucose and olive oil, almond milk can be prepared as we have already mentioned. In addition, the high calcium content and its alkaline pH allow excellent bone mineralization.

Fibre

For more than 40 years, interest in *fibre* in food and its role in reducing the risk of suffering from some diseases has been aroused. Fibre strengthens the immune system, especially known from epidemiological data observed by Dr Denis Burkitt, who died in 1993 at the age of 83 and is recognized worldwide as the father of fibre.[186,187]

Analyzing epidemiological data from around the world and particularly from Africa, where he described what is now known as Burkitt's lymphoma, he remarked that colon cancer was inversely related to the consumption of fibre in the diet.[188,189]

He noted the low incidence compared to the Western world of certain gastrointestinal diseases. This was reversed with the westernization of the diet, by eliminating fibre in refined foods correlated with the increased risk for colorectal cancer, diverticulitis, polyposis, ulcerative colitis, appendicitis and haemorrhoids. The effect of fibre in this regard could be differentiated from that inherent in higher consumption of fruit and vegetables.

For more than 40 years since Burkitt's original description, the observations to date have only reinforced the preventive action of fibre on *colorectal cancer*. The preventive and therapeutic action of fibre on haemorrhoids, hiatal hernia and polyps has also been widely referred to.

It has been questioned whether intestinal diverticulosis is inversely related to fibre consumption, but the observations made show deficiencies in the data collected on eating and defecatory habits prior to the diagnosis of diverticulosis.[190] The effect of fibre in delaying gastric emptying with a slower absorption of nutrients is also evident, which reduces the sudden rise in blood glucose with strong insulin discharges that determine type 2 diabetes. Fibre, because it is resistant to digestion, acts as a prebiotic in the large intestine and favours the development of normal bacterial flora. It constitutes the natural environment, the best one to achieve the development of normal microbiota. Fibre favours the development of the bacillus Bifidus, is bifidogenic and protects against bacterial infections due to shigella and salmonella.

In addition, the fermentation of the fibre by the *intestinal bacterial flora* produces osmotically active substances that retain water, and act like a sponge increasing the volume of the stool, which shortens the intestinal transit time; this has a laxative effect by stimulating intestinal peristalsis, prevents constipation, reduces the contact of faeces with the intestinal epithelium and reduces the concentration of carcinogens.

In the fermentation of fibre, short-chain saturated lipid acids, butyric, propionic, valeric and acetic are originated. Butyric acid that is not present in food constitutes the nutrient par excellence of the colonocyte, a cell of the intestinal epithelium. All these actions are the determinants of a healthy intestine, with a strong immune system, providing protective and preventive action against intestinal and extra-intestinal pathology. It also has anti-inflammatory action and stimulates apoptosis, and programmed cell death, relevant in the control of tumour processes. Fibre is essential for intestinal health, which means structural normality, nutrient-absorbing functional normality and maturing and development as an immune organ with lymphatic structure, defence as a barrier to toxins and bacteria with prevention of infections and chronic intestinal and systemic inflammatory processes.[191,192]

Eating habits with high fibre content reduce the risk of cardiovascular disease and breast cancer, lower the concentration of cholesterol, lipids and glucose in the blood, increase insulin sensitivity, lowers blood pressure and intervene in avoiding weight gain. The fibre present in vegetables is mainly insoluble fibre: cellulose, hemicellulose and lignin, it gives the cells a membrane as a hydrostatic skeleton. In this way, the vegetables, even with up to 95% water maintain their shape and structure. There are soluble fibres such as gums, mucilage and pectin. In most foods that contain fibre, two-thirds of it is insoluble and one-third is soluble.

Although both types of fibre have common activities; the action of soluble fibre can be highlighted in delaying gastric emptying and insoluble fibre combats constipation and prevent polyps and colorectal cancer. The concept of fibre has been expanded to include various compounds with actions similar to those stated, such as indigestible starches or synthetic fibres. They give a feeling of satiety, delay the absorption of simple glucides such as mono and disaccharides, lower blood cholesterol levels by reducing its absorption and have intestinal anti-inflammatory action. Fibre is present in vegetables, both in the pulp and in the membranes, with a certain predominance of those soluble in the pulp and insoluble in the membranes. Sweet potato has a good content of fibre, antioxidants, anthocyanins, beta carotenes and phenolic acid. Reducing the speed of absorption of glucides by fibre avoids sudden and strong insulin discharge, which has a preventive effect on diabetes by reducing blood glucose. It also has a blood cholesterol-lowering action as it decreases intestinal absorption. As one more action on normal intestinal physiology, an association between recurrent abdominal pain and low fibre intake has been observed in children.[193]

There are several beneficial effects of fibre on extraintestinal pathology in addition to the preventive action of diabetes by promoting low glycemic indexes. It prevents obesity due to its positive effect on satiety and low caloric intake. It prevents cardiovascular disease because it promotes the conservation of blood fluidity lowering the concentrations of the plasminogen inhibitor. Plasminogen, as the main fibrinolytic agent, determines the dissolution of clots. In addition, fibre lowers the level of cholesterol in the blood by decreasing its intestinal absorption.[194]

Turmeric has been used since ancient times as a condiment with few systemic effects due to its almost zero solubility and very poor absorption. Mixed with black pepper, due to the action of its active principle piperine, increases its absorption by 2,000% and has beneficial effects on health. Recent studies show that it also behaves like fibre. It has excellent resistance to gastric and intestinal juices, compared to inulin as a standard prebiotic. High-performance liquid chromatography analysis reveals the presence of powerful antioxidants and phenolic curcuminoids and flavonoids and some functional monosaccharides. It is not only digested by lactobacilli and bifid bacteria but also supports the growth of these bacteria and exerts a suppressive effect on the production of interleukin 8 induced by lipopolysaccharides.[195,196]

Regular intake of fibre present in food, by synergistic action with nutrients, has shown not to inhibit minerals and vitamin absorption. The fibre in foods is better than refined fibre processed by the food industry.

A good diet should provide no less than 30 to 40 g. of fibre per day for an adult and 20 to 25g in children 1 to 10 years old. Requirements would appear to be optimal and accurate if we refer to them as 25 to 50g per thousand calories of intake, widely covered by a variety of fruit and vegetables.

The high fibre content of fruit—oranges, papaya and kiwi—and vegetables, such as sweet potatoes should be highlighted.

Meat

Meat, being food from the animal kingdom, together with offal and eggs is one of the main sources of protein intake after the lactation period, due to its high quality and content. It is also a source of vitamin B_{12}, minerals and energy from both structural and storage fats and to a much lesser extent, glucides from liver and muscle glycogen. Cooking meat is best done with water, especially in pressure cookers.

Cooking at high temperatures and low humidity, dry heating in an oven, grilling or frying, should not be part of everyday cooking, because with the

Maillard reaction glycotoxins are produced and absorbed in variable proportions depending on the state of the intestinal epithelium and other factors. The browning of meat should be reserved for occasional meals.

Gelatin from bone broth provides glucosamine, chondroitin sulfate and hyaluronic acid, components of connective tissue that are of fundamental importance for the structural preservation of cartilages, tendons, joints and skin and nails.

The various types of meat, (beef, poultry or pork), are similar in terms of protein and lipid content, while fish and seafood deserve special consideration.

Fish

Fish, especially hake, tuna, salmon, sardines and anchovies, as well as other seafood such as shellfish and seaweed, should be included two or three times a week in our diet. In addition to their protein content, they are special for the quality of their lipids and are rich in omega-3, DHA and EPA.

Salmon should be from the open sea, not from fish farms and it is not recommended for very frequent consumption due to mercury contamination. On the other hand, sardines, anchovies and hake, which are small and shorter-lived and therefore free from significant accumulation of mercury can be eaten frequently along with shellfish and especially krill oil in capsules, available from a pharmacy

Krill

Krill is a small crustacean that abounds in ocean waters. There are several species of different sizes, some 1 to 2cm, others 6 to 12cm. In the southern sea and around the Antarctic, they measure 6cm and weigh 2g. They feed on picoplankton and are food for whales, penguins and fish. They constitute the largest biomass on the planet and are highly sustainable.

They have great nutritional value, especially for their richness in omega-3 lipid acids. Krill oil with its omega-3 contains DHA and EPA like all sea products, unlike omega-3 of vegetable origin, in which only 1 and 3% are converted in the liver into DHA and EPA. In addition, krill oil is available in capsules and has the antioxidant astaxanthin, which is the most powerful antioxidant known, and phospholipids that facilitate its direct entry into cells. This also makes difference with omega-3 of vegetable origin that is unstable and susceptible to oxidation.[197]

Eggs

Eggs are top-quality food. The protein contained in the white is of high biological quality due to its digestibility and absorption and contains all the essential amino acids. The yolk contains lipids and 300 mg. of cholesterol, due to this it was considered to be necessary to limit intake to one egg per week to avoid exceeding 300 mg. of cholesterol per week. But the cholesterol in eggs is metabolized very well, so one egg per day can be eaten. In addition, it has been questioned that cholesterol should be the reason for limitation since there is no evidence that it represents a risk. The so-called bad cholesterol, LDL, is bad when it is oxidized, for this reason, if two eggs are ingested per day, they would have to be subject to minimum cooking.[198,199]

Mushrooms

Fungi include yeasts, moulds and truffles in addition to the better-known English *mushrooms*. Fungi do not have chlorophyll and their cell walls do not have cellulose like plants but rather a chitin-like exoskeleton of arthropods. They do not belong to the plant kingdom, they are closer to the animal kingdom, and they feed on organic material as a source of carbon and energy and as a reserve, glycogen. They are not mobile like animals, nor do they ingest their nutrients, but instead absorb them through fine tubes, underground filaments called hyphae, equivalent to the roots of plants. They are eukaryotes (they have a nucleus, with chromosomes and DNA) different from prokaryotes like bacteria that do not have a nucleus. They have sexual or asexual reproduction. They produce spores that are like seeds. Fungi belong to a separate kingdom, that of fungi, the fungal kingdom. As with plants, there are edible, medicinal and poisonous fungi.

In South America, Argentina was the first country to develop white mushroom crops, mainly in Buenos Aires. The nutritional value of edible mushrooms is in their richness in proteins that make up 19 and 35% of their dry weight, which is less than in meat but more than in vegetables and milk. Taking into account the essential amino acids, the value is similar to meat and milk and higher than pulses and vegetables. They contain the nine essential amino acids, the most abundant of these is lysine, which is the limiting amino acid in cereals. The lowest contents are those of methionine and tryptophan.

They contain all kinds of lipids, from 1.1 to 8.3%, an average of 4%. Seventy-two per cent of the acids are unsaturated, mainly linoleic acid.

They contain between 47 and 81% of glucides, monosaccharides, hexoses and pentoses, oligosaccharides, polysaccharides and glycosides as amino sugars.

The fibre content varies from 4 to 20% and most are not digested or absorbed like glycone, chitin and heteropolysaccharides that absorb toxic substances and accelerate their excretion.

Among the minerals, fungi are rich first in potassium, then in phosphorus, magnesium and sodium, somewhat less in copper and zinc, and even less in iron, manganese, molybdenum, cadmium and calcium. Selenium, which acts synergistically with vitamin E, is found in large quantities in the Agaricus genus, which can be poisonous or edible. Mushrooms which are edible and belong to this genus are high in selenium.

The water content is 70 to 90%.

They are good sources of B_1 (thiamine), B_2 (riboflavin), B_3 (niacin), $B_{7/8}$ (biotin), traces of B_{12} (cobalamin) and D_2 (ergocalciferol). The B_2 content is higher than in vegetables, and B_3, B_7, B_8, B_9 and C are present in moderately high amounts and are higher than in cheese and eggs and are more similar to that of vegetables.

Mushrooms are referred to as beneficial in relation to diseases related to stress and the weakening of the immune system.

Substances derived from fungi have proven immunosuppressive actions and are used for anticancer action in the treatment and prevention. Incorporated regularly in the diet, they also make an important contribution of fibre, calcium, selenium and antioxidants, among which ergothioneine stands out.

Long-chain polysaccharides, particularly alpha and beta-glucan molecules are primarily responsible for the beneficial effect that fungi have on the immune system.[200,201]

With the diet referred to so far, a significant level of endogenous and exogenous antioxidant agents are included, reducing the level of free radicals. To reduce the level of free radicals means reducing cellular damage due to oxidative stress that mainly affects mitochondrial apparatus reducing energy generation. In this way, the ageing process is slowed down, which has been called the antiageing action, and cognitive functions are preserved.

CHAPTER 4

METABOLIC ALTERATION IN NUTRITIONAL DISEASES

Weight gain and obesity

Weight gain and *obesity* to various degrees constitute an endemic problem in developed and developing countries. Weight gain affects more than 60% and obesity affects more than 20% of the population, even in childhood the percentages are increasing, thus configuring what can be considered the epidemic of the century, which could be referred to by the term ‘globesity’. The severity of this problem derives, in addition to the decrease in quality of life, from the increased risk of mortality among other causes due to metabolic complications, diabetes and cardiovascular disease.

Since the discovery of adipokines, hormones secreted by adipose tissue, it is considered an endocrine organ with an important influence on the regulation of appetite, satiety, thermogenesis, energy expenditure, insulin sensitivity and secretion, glucides and lipids metabolism, fat distribution, blood pressure and immune system function.

Subcutaneous connective tissue and its adipose filling as an endocrine organ secrete hormones called *adipokines*, which are specific cytokines secreted by adipocytes, such as leptin stimulated by insulin with anorexigenic action which decreases appetite, and *adiponectin* with its anti-inflammatory action, and both increase insulin sensitivity.

In contrast to the normal structure of connective tissue, with adipocytes, preadipocytes and few leukocytes, in obesity fibroblasts, neutrophils, monocytes, T lymphocytes and hypertrophy of adipocytes with hypoxia due to less flow and areas of necrosis, are observed. *Leptin* secretion increases with peripheral resistance and decreases adiponectin secretion with the consequent increase in *insulin resistance* and fatty liver is generated with metabolic syndrome, with the low-grade chronic inflammatory processes6, CRP and TNF-alpha increased.

Muscles normally make between 40 and 50% of body mass and together with fat are the main consumers of glucose and for this they need insulin.

Resveratrol, curcumin, taurine and circumine improve the response to insulin with a hypoglycemic effect.[202-204]

The ready availability of white sugar, or HFCS that have largely displaced white sugar in baking, contributes to addictive 'hollow' calories, leading to weight gain and obesity. To this is added the aggravating factor that since sugar is a glucid with a high glycemic index, it determines strong insulin discharges, which favours the development of insulin resistance and thus the production of type 2 diabetes. In addition, vitamins B_3, B_5, B_6 and B_{12}, the amino acids tryptophan and methionine, and minerals are used to metabolize glucose-fructose syrup or powder, although it has been argued that since it does not require insulin for metabolism, it does not promote diabetes, but it has a potentiating effect on weight gain and obesity. The intake of fructose and the lower insulin discharge decreases the release of leptin and the appetite is not inhibited.

On the other hand, the gastric mucosa secretes ghrelin, an orexigenic hormone, that stimulates the appetite. In the postprandial period, there is a drop in ghrelin secretion and this drop is less with fructose ingestion. These two secondary actions of fructose; lower leptin release and insufficient postprandial drop in ghrelin, lead to increased intake, leading to weight gain and obesity.

Glucose is metabolized in all cells of the body, but fructose is metabolized in the liver for the synthesis of glycogen as an energy reserve and the excess is metabolized creating uric acid as the final product.[205-208]

People who do not gain weight can also have metabolic syndrome. One in four thin people have insulin resistance, with blood glucose between 100 and 125mg%, and they are pre-diabetic or type 2 diabetic. These patients are thin/obese because they have a greater amount of fat in relation to their muscle mass.

An increase in body fat is a contributing factor to low levels of *Vitamin D* (25 OH cholecalciferol) since this vitamin is fat-soluble and is trapped in the fatty tissue, therefore vitamin D supplement is required since its deficit is also a cause of insulin resistance.

There is not necessarily a correlation between weight gain or obesity and metabolic syndrome, the body mass index is greater with a normal metabolic picture, and a body mass index of less than 25 with metabolic syndrome. The *body mass index* is not a faithful parameter of metabolic health, as it is the insulin level. A more faithful parameter may be the abdominal circumference. Measurement of the abdominal circumference is independent and complementary to the body mass index to predict the health risk at any age.[209-214]

Optimal *abdominal circumference* for health in men can be considered from 80 to 95 cm, greater than 95 already implies risk, which is high if it exceeds 102 cm. For women, an optimal value would be 70 to 82cm: greater than 82 would imply risk, which becomes high if it exceeds 88 cm.

Simply, we can appreciate the thickness of the vertical fold of the skin of the abdomen taken between the index and thumb. The optimum is 1cm, and tolerable up to 2 cm.

Leptin, adiponectin and pro-inflammatory cytokines are the main hormones under study. Leptin is anorectic, and adiponectin is anti-inflammatory and anti-apoptotic. Both increase insulin sensitivity and are stimulated by insulin and its actions, which are broader and more complex, and these are being studied, as well as therapeutic applications.[215-217]

For several decades now, given the alarming increase in weight gain and obesity, weight-loss diets are the ones that have proliferated the most. Many of these diets aiming to reduce caloric intake pay special attention only to the quantitative aspect, limiting the size of the servings. All programs implemented solely on the basis of caloric restriction have demonstrated their failure, which is evidenced in the continuous increase of this pathology with the follow-up of patients in the medium and long term.

Hypocaloric diets focused on the specific objective of losing weight are not the most convenient for achieving a state of health, and their follow-up in most cases is carried out for a limited time. These diets can even be inconvenient because losing weight without improving health can lead to further deterioration, such as osteoporotic fractures from minor trauma by losing the protection of the adipose lining. On the other hand, especially in women who are not obese or even overweight, it is relatively frequent that they follow low-calorie diets, especially before summer, for aesthetic reasons based on subjective distortions of their body image. The best way to correct variable forms and degrees of obesity or weight gain is optimal meals to improve health, as referred to in Chapter 2.

Patients affected by weight gain or obesity, during their medical care, in addition to food and nutritional control, require guidance on aerobic physical activities, in many cases psychological support and sometimes drug treatment. Extreme cases of obesity that interfere with normal life and present metabolic problems are subject to surgery, such as bariatric surgery.

Surgery for obesity uses restrictive techniques and malabsorptive techniques. Restrictive techniques, such as partial, tubular or vertical gastrectomy, limit the amount of food that can be eaten and delay gastric evacuation, increasing the feeling of satiety. Malabsorptive techniques, with a gastrointestinal bypass, decrease the absorption of fats and, to a lesser extent, proteins. In the follow-up of these patients, post-surgery diets with the control of possible complications and supplementation of vitamins and minerals are essential to avoid nutritional deficiencies, especially in malabsorptive techniques. Obesity is a multifactorial problem, where genetics also intervenes but in no more than 10% of cases and can always be prevented through healthy lifestyle habits. For the prevention of weight gain and obesity, together with physical activity and avoiding a sedentary lifestyle, healthy eating behaviour is fundamental, prioritizing quality rather than quantity of food.

Hyperuricemia

Both common sugar and HFCS have a high glycemic index, adding an unwanted caloric intake, and *hyperuricemia* decrease levels of nitric oxide which makes it difficult for glucose to enter cells, thereby generating insulin resistance. Hyperuricemia can create uric acid deposits, tophi, in distal joints, mainly of the big toe with very painful arthritis that leads to *gout*. Arthritis can also affect the joints of other fingers or the knees, arthritis that can lead to osteoarthritis. Hyperuricemia can also cause urinary stones and kidney damage. Apigenin, a bioflavonoid contained in celery, parsley, thyme and onions, inhibits xanthine oxidase that transforms purines into uric acid. Allopurinol, a medication used in patients with hyperuricemia, has the same action. Also, vitamin C decreases uricemia levels.

Insulin resistance. Type 2 diabetes

Both sucrose and HFCS are artificial products that are very easy and fast to absorb. They do not exist in nature in that isolated ‘pure’ form, without other nutrients. They are net glucides, 'bad' glucides because they have no overall nutritional value as food; their ingestion means nothing more than a contribution of 'hollow' calories. The rapid absorption of sugar and fructose syrup, whether from processed foods, such as ice cream, desserts or sweets or that we incorporate at the table, has a high glycemic index and a high glycemic load. This determines sharp elevations in insulin discharges.

Metabolic syndrome

The ingestion of sugar or fructose syrup in the usual diet has deleterious effects on health, weight gain or obesity, insulin resistance, *type 2 diabetes* and *metabolic syndrome*, which are potentiated by other alterations in eating behaviour and sedentary life.

With the diagnostic criteria of the WHO or NCEP,[218,219] metabolic syndrome, syndrome X, may be integrated by:

- Waist circumference greater than 102 cm in men and 88 cm. in women.
- Increase in *triglycerides*: greater than 150mg%.
- Good cholesterol or *HDL is* less than 40mg% in men and 50 mg% in women according to NCEP.
- Fasting blood glucose greater than 110mg%, according to NCEP.
- *Microalbuminuria* (urinary albumin excretion) greater than 20mg/L.
- *Blood pressure* greater than 135/85 according to NCEP or 139/89 according to WHO.

Cinnamon has shown benefits for the control of metabolic disorders of type 2 diabetes, with decreased blood glucose, increased HDL and decreased LDL and triglycerides. No decreases in glycated haemoglobin were seen, but the necessary doses and the required follow-up times have not been specified.[220]

Statins, used as cholesterol-lowering drugs, can have adverse effects, such as muscle disorders due to rhabdomyolysis, alteration of the structure of muscle fibres, sarcopenia, loss of muscle mass, muscle aches and fatigue. There may also be alterations in liver and mitochondria function with the consequent detriment in energy performance.[221]

Seventy-five per cent of cholesterol is produced in the liver and is an important precursor compound for the synthesis of vitamin D and the hormones cortisol, estrogens and progesterone and promotes digestion as a component of bile. Consequently, cholesterol is present in foods of animal origin, but its production in the liver is also stimulated by high levels of insulin in type 2 diabetes. Contrary to this, a normal level of cholesterol is favoured by vitamin D.

High levels of total cholesterol at the expense of the so-called bad cholesterol or LDL is referred to as a conditioning factor for arteriosclerosis, but cholesterol is bad when it is oxidized and plasma cholesterol levels can be corrected with control of the metabolic imbalance. Also, the carotenoids of fruit and vegetables, lycopene and other phytochemicals prevent the oxidation of cholesterol and help to maintain normal levels. Levels of total LDL and HDL cholesterol below normal could be risk factors for certain types of cancer.

An optimal diet is a better resource to normalize cholesterol than statins.

Blood glucose may be normal because to compensate for insulin resistance, the pancreas increases the secretion of this hormone. This is evidenced by an increase in the level of insulin in plasma whose normal value is up to 8.8 uIU/ml. in men and 8.4 in women, but for people with a low intake of processed foods, such as pasta and sweets, it is less than 2. Insulin resistance is more accurately diagnosed with the *HOMA* index, which stands for homeostasis model assessment, using the formula to quantify insulin resistance. A value greater than 3 has a 90% chance of corresponding to insulin resistance[222,223.]

$$\text{HOMA} = \frac{\text{Blood glucose (mg\%)} \times \text{insulin (uIU/ml)}}{405}.$$

Hyperinsulinemia enhanced by lipokines such as TNFα and IL6 produced by adipocytes that act as an endocrine organ is a promoter of inflammation and oxidative stress, a high-risk factor for increased fat in the liver; non-alcoholic hepatic steatosis that can lead to cirrhosis. Insulin transports fat to deposits, lipogenesis and inhibits lipolysis. Insulin lowers during fasting and facilitates fat mobilization.

Resveratrol, quercetin and cinnamon, among other antioxidant and anti-inflammatory active ingredients of various herbs, have preventive action in regular nutrition. Extracts that can be dosed for therapeutic actions are being studied[224,225].

Type 3 diabetes and Alzheimer's disease

The pathogenic line of insulin resistance, which is seen as a consequence of weight gain and obesity and which generates type 2 diabetes with metabolic syndrome, in recent years has been linked to *Alzheimer's disease*. In autopsies of patients with Alzheimer's disease, low levels of insulin were found in the affected areas; the frontal cortex, hippocampus and hypothalamus, with neuritic plaques due to amyloid-like protein deposits and the formation of amyloid fibres and neuronal loss. This does not occur in unaffected areas such as the cerebellum.

Abnormalities in response to insulin and insulin growth factors I and II and low levels of insulin receptors at the brain level, alteration in the energy metabolism of mitochondrial function, oxidative stress and reduced glucose utilization, characterize Alzheimer's disease as a neuroendocrine disorder that resembles a distinct form of diabetes, type 3 diabetes.[226-230]

Even today, in addition to proteins, lipids, glucides, vitamins and minerals, which the food and pharmaceutical industry has isolated and offered in a pure form, there are many other macro and micronutrient substances such as antioxidants, flavonoids, and even vitamins not yet known, and innumerable macro and microelements present in natural foods with variable chemical structures that act in synergistic actions that are still little known.

Sucrose and fructose, in nature, are found together with other simple and complex glucides, oligosaccharides and reserve or structural polysaccharides, many of the latter as fibres. All in synergic functions with vitamins, enzymes and minerals.

In our meals, vegetables and fruit in a natural state have a low glycemic index and a high water content; between 85 and 95% determines a low glycemic load. The slow absorption of glucides due to the presence of fibre makes the increases in blood glucose after their intake significantly lower than that resulting from the ingestion of processed foods, with high energy density, due to their low water content.

The pathogenic role of glycotoxins

Cooking some foods at high temperatures, 130ºC-170ºC in the oven, grilling or frying triggers complex chemical reactions called *glycation* as described by the French doctor and chemist, Louis Camille Maillard in 1912.[231] Glycation determines colour, aroma and flavour changes, which make foods such as meat, bread and French fries particularly palatable.[232] This is why glycation, or the *Maillard reaction,* has been an object of interest in gastronomy. The colour changes, typical of toasting, are due to brown compounds called melanoidins. The intensity of food glycation is strongly accelerated at high temperatures with low humidity, such as dry heat in the aforementioned cooking methods, and is facilitated by iron and copper in the cooking utensils and by alkaline media. By cooking in the above-mentioned way, some foods such as bakery products, (bread, cakes or biscuits) can cause a true addiction, becoming a determinant of weight gain and obesity.

Caramel, which is made by the prolonged boiling of condensed milk, has its brownish colour mainly due to caramelization, but the one made for confectionery has a brownish colour which is more intense due to the glycation facilitated by the addition of sodium bicarbonate.

Opposite to this confectionery, the addition of acidity, using lemon juice, to meat, bread or potatoes before cooking attenuates the glycation. *Glycation* consists of the non-enzymatic union of the carbonyl group(C = OH) of reducing sugars such as glucose and fructose with the amino group (NH_2) of proteins and nucleic acids with changes in chemical structure and function. Carbonyl groups also originate with lipid-oxidative degradation. Since the description of glycation during cooking under referred conditions, *exogenous glycation*, more than 60 years elapsed until 1976 when an increasing interest in physiology observed that a fraction of haemoglobin increased in diabetic patients[233] is in glycated form, *glycated haemoglobin* (Hb_{1c}), misnamed *glycosylated haemoglobin.*

E*ndogenous glycation* in the extracellular correlates with the level of glycemia, while in the intracellular is correlated with the products of glucose metabolization and especially with fructose that freely enters the cells and is more reactive than glucose. *Fructose* does not intervene in extracellular glycation since its concentration is scarcely 1% of glycemia. In addition to the exogenous glycation that occurs during food cooking, in the last decade glycation has been reported in situ, in the intestinal lumen when ingesting apple juice together with egg albumin. This is also exogenous glycation as it occurs in the intestinal lumen, not in the internal, extra or intracellular environment.[234,235] Exogenous glycation products are excreted by faecal matter and are partially absorbed depending on the type of diet and integrity of the intestinal epithelium, largely dependent on the state of the intestinal microbiota.

Among the compounds resulting from glycation are the so-called *advanced glycation products* (AGPs) that are generators of free radicals and promoters of inflammation, which can mean damage to vessels and parenchyma.

In *endogenous glycation*, the proteins most affected are those with the longest half-life, less renewal or turnover.

Proteins of the retina, lens, kidneys, connective tissue, myelin and basement membranes of blood vessels, all of which have a long half-life, can be transformed into glycation products and accumulate for years in arterial walls and basement membranes of capillaries. Glycation is controlled by inhibitors of the initial glycation products, antioxidants and anti-inflammatories of the organism and is also present to a great extent in natural foods. Glycation products can play a pathogenic role in ageing and chronic kidney failure, due to lower antioxidant activity and reduced elimination, and in diabetes, due to higher blood glucose levels. Excess glycation is a major aggravating risk factor in diabetes, chronic kidney failure and chronic obstructive pulmonary disease. It can also play pathogenic roles in early ageing, especially in skin and vascular endothelium, cardiovascular disease, brain deterioration and neurodegenerative diseases.[236-238] Glycated proteins are denatured proteins, with amino acids that have lost their normal three-dimensional conformation, which alters their actions with potentially adverse effects on health, promoting inflammatory processes.[239,240]

The accumulation of AGPs in tissues over the years is involved in the pathological process of diseases such as cataracts, glomerulosclerosis and atherosclerosis. As a relevant factor in the ageing process, it is especially evident in the evolution of diabetes with the development of the three well-known secondary pathologies: nephropathy, retinopathy and diabetic neuropathy. Within cells, the consequent damage to AGPs occurs especially in the mitochondria, decreasing energy production. In tissues with short half-life proteins, due to a more active cell renewal process, such as the intestine, skin and liver, the damage occurs mainly in the DNA, being the cause of mutations, deletions and insertions, potentially carcinogenic. Also acrylamide and furan, by-products of the Maillard reaction are carcinogenic substances. In Alzheimer's disease, AGPs in beta-amyloid plaques are observed at three times higher than in controls. Due to the glycation of proteins, it has been observed as affected enzymes, with a decrease in their activity, to calmodulin, superoxide dismutase and Ca^{++}-ATPase and with an increase in activity to aldose reductase. The alteration in superoxide dismutase function increases the harmful effect of free radicals, while the affectation of calmodulin and Ca^{++}-ATPase (of the calcium pump) increase intracellular calcium concentration, with effects on muscle contraction, gene expression, cell differentiation and neuronal functions. Increased aldose reductase activity produces fructose from glucose.[241]

Glycated haemoglobin

The level of AGPs generated in the body is related to the level of glycemia. In chronic hyperglycemia such as prediabetics and diabetics, the structural alteration of haemoglobin, glycated haemoglobin (HbA_{1c}), occurs. The normal level of HbA_{1c} in non-diabetics is between 4.2 and 5.8% and in diabetics, with good control of their disease, it should not exceed 7.6% which corresponds to fasting glucose of 125 mg%. Untreated diabetics can show HbA_{1c}levels as high as 20mg%. The measurement of HbA_{1c} is more representative of the control of treatment in diabetes than isolated measurements of fasting blood glucose. Glycated haemoglobin values represent the average blood glucose for the three or four weeks prior to the study. However, HbA_{1c} does not allow for detecting specific drops or rises in blood glucose as serial blood glucose measurements. Both haemoglobin and proteins in the lens, retina and connective tissue are among the most vulnerable to glycation. The term glycosylated haemoglobin used generally is incorrect, it must be glycated haemoglobin because it is nothing more than the glycation of haemoglobin produced by glucose in the blood. *Glycosylation* is always enzymatic, physiological and highly controlled and occurs in proteins after gene transcription and modulates their function. Glycation is non-enzymatic; therefore some authors refer to it as non-enzymatic glycosylation, but that does not exist; glycation and glycosylation are two different chemical processes.[242]

An excessive level of AGPs increases the generation of free radicals and cytokines that promote inflammatory processes with organic damage to the liver, kidney, blood vessels, the brain, lenses, the retina and the connective tissue of the skin, cartilage and tendons.

Glycation products, because they have potentially adverse health effects, are also called glycotoxins and are the cause of damage to various organs. Damage caused by glycotoxins is seen in the fatty liver that can lead to cirrhosis similar to that observed in chronic alcoholism, in the kidneys with glomeruli basement membrane thickening, in blood vessels with deposits of atheroma plaques, in the brain with a deposit of beta-amyloid plaques observable in Alzheimer's disease, in connective tissue accelerating skin ageing and giving rigidity of cartilage and tendons and in the crystalline lens causing cataracts.

The decrease in brain volume observed in some subjects in the course of ageing, among other factors, has been related to HbA_{1c} levels.[243]

In children with type 1 diabetes treated at the Elizalde Hospital in Buenos Aires and who were monitored in the Nephrology service for their renal function, joint stiffness in the hands was observed in addition to retinopathy and nephropathy. This is called the Rosenbloom's sign and because of its obviousness and simplicity, it constitutes a valuable part of the semiological picture. Alteration by glycation of the structural proteins in the connective tissue of tendons and cartilage is the cause of stiffness that limits joint movements.

Joint stiffness can be recorded on the palmar impression, compared to controls.

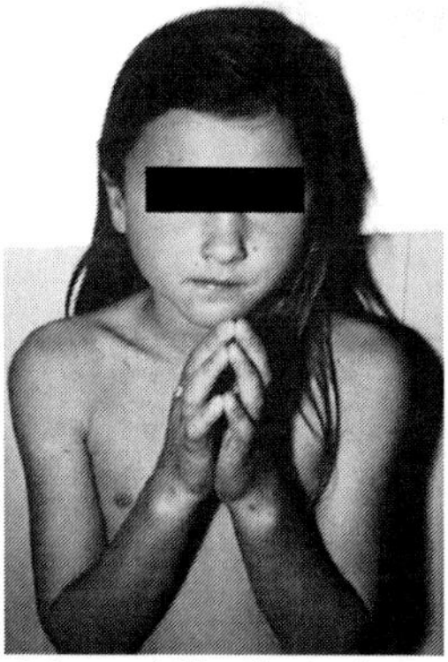
Joint mobility limitation

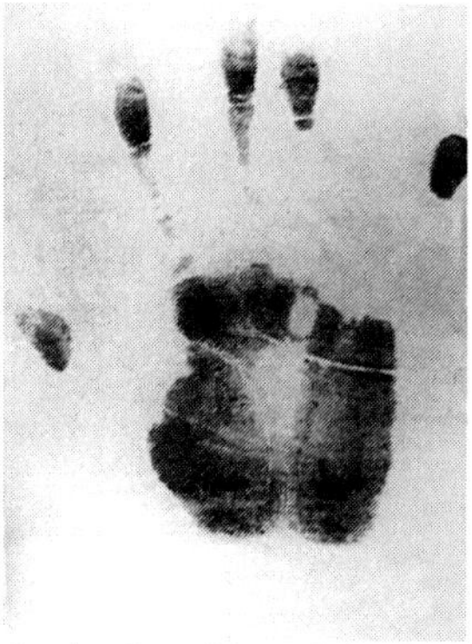
Lack of marking of the first phalanges

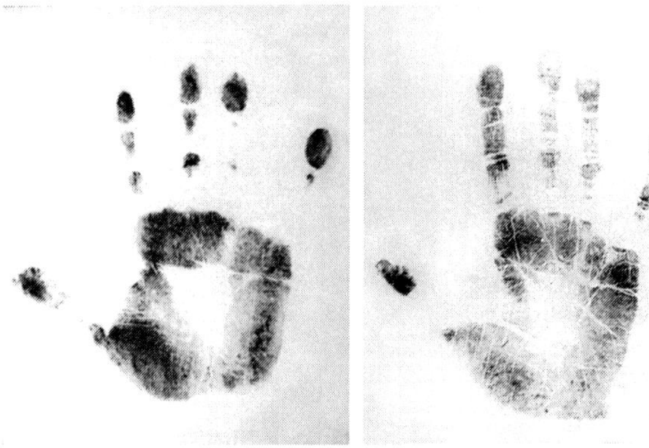

Diabetics without kidney disease Normal control

Photo 4-1: Diabetic nephropathy patient

In *diabetic nephropathy*, after the first stage of functional alterations, the second stage of structural alterations is characterized by thickening of the basement membrane, expansion of connective tissue, the mesangium and changes in the glomerular arteries. Immunological participation has not been documented in these lesions and an alteration of the structural proteins seems to be the main pathogenic factor[244, 245.]

Clinical observations and animal experiments show that cooking foods at high temperatures in dry heat and a high fructose intake are important risk factors in diabetic Mellitus, cardiovascular disease, neurodegenerative and other age-related diseases.[246,247]

A study carried out on normal, non-diabetic subjects after ingestion of foods cooked at high temperatures did not show increases or decreases of AGPs in plasma or urine.[248] The production and absorption of these products possibly vary according to the presence of antioxidants, the state of the intestinal epithelium and the quality of the microbiota. Other studies show decreased insulin sensitivity, decreased levels of omega-3 lipid acids, vitamins C and E and increased cholesterol and triglycerides.[249]

AGP inhibitory agents are being evaluated for clinical use.[250]

Glycation also affects nucleic acids, which can alter DNA.

Poorly controlled diabetic mothers during pregnancy can give rise to children with congenital malformations, as we saw in patients with caudal retraction sequence, with the mildest form being sacral agenesis or the most severe, syringomyelia or sympathetic fusion of the buds of lower limbs. These malformations are the consequence of a defect of the caudal blastema or the posterior middle portion of the mesoderm; we do not know if they are due to alteration of the structural proteins of the connective tissue or are secondary to nucleic acid alterations.[251]

Reducing AGPs is relevant not only in diabetes but also in patients with chronic renal failure, with reduced elimination of carbonyl groups that are highly reactive to glycation. The reduction of AGPs in patients with advanced chronic renal failure allows better clinical and humoral evolution. AGPs are fluorescent, which determines an increase in fluorescence in the skin in subjects according to the degree of skin ageing. This has also been referred to as an index of vascular and renal damage and prognostic value in patients on hemodialysis or with kidney transplantation.[252-254] A decrease in AGPs of food origin through changes in culinary technology not only could decrease the levels of these glycotoxins in serum but also decreases the markers of oxidative stress and inflammation. This provides undoubted benefits in the evolution of patients with states of advanced chronic renal failure.[255]

Increased accumulation of AGPs has been associated with end-stage renal disease, chronic obstructive pulmonary disease and the ageing process. For factors that influence the ageing process, the skin is considered an important study organ. Skin is an important barrier between the body and the external environment; this exposes it to a series of factors that make it especially vulnerable and depends on the preservation of its integrity of nutrition and immunological mechanisms and these factors are closely related.

Endogenously generated ability to decrease AGPs has been attributed to various herbs and spices, such as cinnamon, cloves, oregano, ginger and garlic. This capacity has been attributed to various compounds such as alpha lipoic acid, carnitine, taurine, carnosine, benfotiamine, alpha-tocopherol, niacinamide, pyridoxal, riboflavin or elements such as selenium, zinc or manganese.[256,257] Theoretically, as the generation of AGPs is accelerated by reactive oxygen species, antioxidants, such as resveratrol, present in wine, (especially in red wine) on which some studies have been made, would be effective in limiting its production.[258, 259] Through fluorescence, a decrease in AGPs as a result of sport has been observed.[260]

More studies are needed to be able to add with certainty other benefits in relation to the ageing process to what has been until now indisputable:

restricting caloric intake and controlling blood glucose avoiding net glucides, that is without fibre, the fructose and sucrose present mainly in processed and ultra-processed foods and replacing net glucides with fibre present in natural foods, vegetables and fruit.[261,262]

Glycation products are of exogenous and endogenous origin.

Exogenous production corresponds to the diet, which in relation to AGPs are referred to as dAGPs. They are generated mainly during the manufacture of food subjected to high temperatures with low humidity; dry heat.

Glycation products of food origin are absorbed in a variable percentage that can reach up to 30% according to the state of intestinal health depending on the microbiota. The main nutrient of the intestinal epithelium is butyric acid produced by intestinal flora from the fermentation of dietary fibre. Also of high importance are the microbiome, metabolites and nucleic acids of the microbiota and of nutritional origin whose enzymes allow the hydrolysis necessary for the absorption of antioxidants and sequestering action of AGPs. The absorbed AGPs are partially inactivated and excreted, and depending on nutritional and metabolic variables they are also retained in various organs and tissues. Glycation of endogenous origin occurs in small amounts during metabolism under physiological conditions, both extra and intracellular. In the extracellular, it results from the interaction of glucose with plasma proteins and lipids. In the intracellular glucose metabolites such as glucose-6-phosphate and glyceraldehyde-3-phosphate react strongly with their free carbonyl groups, against proteins, lipids and nucleic acids. This occurs not only in the cytoplasm but also in the mitochondria, the largest cellular organelle's main producers of energy.

Elevated blood glucose and a high intake of dAGPs increases endogenous glycation.

Consumption of alcohol in excess, through its metabolite acetaldehyde and also dark beer and sugar-rich alcohol, can be important contributors to the generation of AGPs.

Glycation products can be measured in blood, urine and tissues by various methods. In the skin, they can be detected by autofluorescence. Of the hundreds of AGPs that are already known, one of the most prevalent, *carboxymethyl lysine* is almost absent in areas of the body with sun protection, it is postulated that UV rays can mediate its formation or make cells more sensitive for fixing. Glycation products are partially inactivated inside and outside cells and excreted in the urine.

The simultaneous ingestion of alcohol and fruit favours AGP production, as the liver metabolizes alcohol and increases the concentration of fructose in the intra and extracellular and fructose is more reactive than glucose. Fat and muscles are the main consumers of glucose; in diabetes due to insulin resistance or deficiency they cannot use it and then the other tissues that do not need insulin have glucose in the intra and extracellular.

Special damage is observed in those with diabetes and chronic kidney disease and the elderly because they do not eliminate highly reactive carbonylic compounds (carbonyl stress) in DNA. Its low turnover leads to chromosomal alterations and impaired replication, repair and transcription.

AGPs are inducers of apoptosis that are usually used to replace damaged or developing cells.

The theory of ageing is of a deleterious network in which oxidative stress, free radicals and mitochondrial damage participate, in all of which glycation participates.[263]

AGPs preforms as a result of high-temperature cooking in contrast to steaming or boiling. A low

dAGP shows low levels of inflammatory markers such as IL6, TNFα, and CRP. Mitochondrial dysfunction has been postulated as an intervening factor in schizophrenia, bipolar disorder, Alzheimer's disease, Parkinson's disease, epilepsy, migraine, cardiovascular disease, cardiomyopathy including heart attacks, ataxia, chronic fatigue syndrome, retinitis pigmentosa, diabetes, hepatitis C, primary biliary cirrhosis and lately its role in carcinogenesis is being studied. Glycation originates from cooking and also plays a pathogenic role in food allergy and its inflammatory processes.[264,265]

Attenuating the potential pathogenic effects of glycotoxins

Based on all the aforementioned measures, reducing the intake of certain foods (without completely banning them) for occasional but not daily consumption, plus lifestyle changes can contribute successfully to *health preservation.* Table 4-1.

The Attenuating potential pathogenic effects of glycotoxins
Alimentary habits and lifestyle

- Give a preference to boiling, steaming or microwaving for cooking
- Use lemon juice or vinegar acidification before grilling, on the griddle or oven
- Avoid foods with a high glycemic index
- Avoid sugar, glucose and fructose, especially in processed foods and soft drinks
- Eat daily 2 or 3 portions of fresh vegetables and fruits
- Use spices: turmeric, ginger, cinnamon, clove and black pepper
- Consume tea and Yerba Mate
- Drink red wine, one glass daily
- Exercise or do sport 5 days a week
- Limit alcohol consumption. Quit smoking
- Avoid foods with low nutritional value and high caloric density

Table 4-1
From: Voyer LE, Alvarado C.[242.]

Cancer and diet

With the treatment of *cancer* using chemotherapy, immune or radiotherapy and surgery, the success achieved in most cases, especially with early diagnosis, in terms of prolonged survival in good conditions is notable. However, in many cases, after many years of control, reactivations and metastases are observed, some also of a long evolution, such as bone metastases or the more serious visceral metastases.

Mitochondrial metabolism

In the last decade, the metabolic theory of cancer has taken effect, enunciated by Otto Warburg, Nobel Prize winner in 1931 and postulated for a second Nobel in 1944.[266-268]

According to the theory of symbiotic evolution on the origin of mitochondria, which continues to be the subject of interesting studies, between one and three billion years ago, eukaryotic cells, (where DNA is condensed in the nuclei forming chromosomes), incorporated by endocytosis prokaryotic organisms, (without nuclei where DNA is dispersed in the cytoplasm), similar to aerobic bacteria, became mitochondria.[269-272] (Fig. 4-1) Mitochondria generate energy in exchange for double-membrane protection and a secure supply of nutrients. In this way, a symbiosis is constituted, a way of life characterized by the close relationship of organisms of different species, generally with mutual benefit.

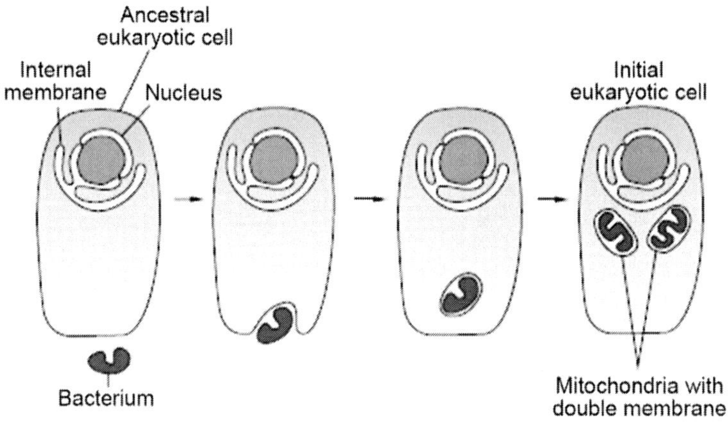

Fig. 4-1: Evolution from ancestral eukaryotic cells to mitochondrial integration

Mitochondria, the largest subcellular corpuscles or organelles, have been referred to as conductors in cellular metabolism. With their high oxygen consumption and strongly aerobic metabolism, they are of fundamental importance for energy production and the regulation of *apoptosis* (programmed cell death). Apoptosis is essential for the preservation of health; it allows the regular replacement of 30 to 50 trillion cells per day and the compounds derived from apoptosis are reused by the cells. Different from apoptosis is necrosis, pathological cell death secondary to injury, which causes the release of waste compounds that are the cause of inflammation and acidosis. Autolysis, which is cell death due to enzymatic actions, as occurs in acute pancreatitis, is also different.

Mitochondria normally supply between 90 and 95% of cellular energy by oxidative phosphorylation coupled to aerobic glycolysis in the electron transport chain of the Krebs cycle, or tricarboxylic acid cycle, with production per gram molecule (mole) of glucose, 38 molecules of adenosine-tri-phosphate (ATP) and as final metabolic products, carbonic anhydride and water.

Evolution from ancestral eukaryotic cell to mitochondrial integration

Only between 5 and 10% of the energy is generated in the cytoplasm, with little oxygen availability, also called glucose fermentation, (the Pasteur Meyerhof cycle), with the production for each mole of glucose of only 2 molecules of ATP, with lactic acid as the final product.

The metabolic intensity of a cell is determined by the number of mitochondria it contains, which varies from hundreds to thousands. The highest amounts are found in the brain (with 25% of the total energy expenditure) muscles, the liver and heart.[273,274] Mitochondrial functionalism with energy production, regulation of apoptosis and cell metabolism decreases with biological age, conditioned not only by chronological age but also by epigenetic factors such as habit, diet and environmental factors.

Adverse biological circumstances such as a sedentary lifestyle, drug addiction, smoking, malnutrition, obesity and psychological stress, abusive use of xenobiotics as NSAIDs psychotropics, antibiotics, hypoglycemic agents, hypocholesterolemic agents, anticonvulsants, pesticides, insecticides, inflammatory processes and chronic conditions harmful to cell structure and function and mainly to mitochondrial energy metabolism, by the action on DNA or directly on enzymatic actions, produce depletion of energy metabolism.[275,276]

The American Food and Drug Administration does not yet impose toxicity controls on the mitochondria for pharmaceutical products.

Xenobiotics also have other risks that generally outweigh the benefits.

Nonsteroidal anti-inflammatory pain relievers in early pregnancy double the risk of loss.[277]

Antiperspirants contain aluminium that alters normal bacterial flora replaced by odour-causing actinobacteria and the risk of cancer and Alzheimer's disease is being studied in relation to this.[278]

The regular use of pain relievers, aspirin, acetaminophen and NSAIDs increases the risk of hearing loss in young men, especially those under 50 years of age.[279] In our work on salicylic intoxication, in complementary studies we have demonstrated in vitro with slices of the renal cortex, the inhibitory effect of salicylates on gluconeogenesis.[280, 281]

Unlike nuclear DNA, mitochondrial DNA lacks histones, proteins that coat DNA and preserve its integrity by protecting it from various damaging agents. Histone deficiency makes mitochondrial DNA vulnerable, and susceptible to damage, mainly by free radicals.

With *mitochondrial dysfunction,* its energy production decreases, which can reach less than 50%, which leads to an increase in cytoplasmic glycolysis, with lower energy generation and the high production of lactic acid, lactic acidemia acidosis, which further interferes with mitochondrial function, activates angiogenesis (generation of new blood vessels) and degradation of the cell-matrix, which facilitates tumour growth and spread.[268,282, 283]

Only 2 ATP is produced for each mole of glucose in the cytoplasm instead of 38 ATP for each mole of glucose generated in the mitochondria.[284,285] This regression to an archaic metabolism model occurs as an adaptation to adverse biological conditions. Acrylamide and furan, by-products of the Maillard reaction, are also carcinogenic risk factors over time. Numerous observations between 2013 and 2017 make evident the pathogenic role of high fructose consumption in the generation of AGPs. This makes precautionary measures necessary not only for the consumption of sucrose, which is common sugar but also for fructose, which should be limited to the content of 200 or 400g of fruit per day.

Until 1970, *fructose consumption* was 6 to 12g per day corresponding to the content of the fruit. Later limitations in the availability and the high cost of sugar led to the use of fructose from HFCS as an alternative in gastronomy. Consequently, fructose consumption has increased considerably since 1980 through numerous processed and ultra-processed foods.

Strong epidemiological data show diabetics at increased risk for some types of cancer such as pancreas, liver, stomach, endometrium, as well as colorectal, urinary and breast cancer. Likewise, it has been observed that diabetic patients with cancer have a worse prognosis after chemotherapy or surgery. The direct relationship between glycated haemoglobin and cancer has been observed not only in diabetics but also in normal subjects. This has led to the postulation of new therapeutic approaches currently under study.[286-290] Due to the depletion of apoptosis as a consequence of mitochondrial dysfunction, there is an uncontrolled proliferation of cells, which together with lactic acidemia acidosis that activates angiogenesis and the degradation of the cell matrix, facilitates the growth and spread of the tumour.[291-294] In this situation, cancer may arise as a consequence of dysbiosis between mitochondrial and cytoplasmic metabolism, as an adaptive mechanism to adverse biological circumstances.[295] In cancer, most cells have a highly glucose-dependent metabolism, as mitochondrial dysfunction hinders the metabolism of lipid acids and ketone bodies. High levels of insulin and insulin growth factors favour cell proliferation, angiogenesis and antiapoptotic activity.

Glucose restriction strongly limits cancer development favouring cell death.[296,297]

A*cid-base imbalance* also intervenes in carcinogenesis, since the acidosis that can occur due to an acidic diet interferes with the absorption of oxygen, while an alkaline diet favours aerobic metabolism. Blood pH above 7.4 prevents mitochondrial damage, while pH at its lower limit, 7.35, a state close to acidosis causes a deterioration of mitochondrial function. An alkaline diet with a predominance of fruit and vegetables and not an acidic diet of meat, cereals and pulses is an important determinant of mitochondrial health. The alkaline diet favours oxygen absorption and the reverse, the acidic diet, releases it. In addition to the benefit of an alkaline diet in the treatment of cancer, studies have been carried out on alternative therapies such as hyperbaric oxygenation on the one hand and antioxidants together with ketogenic diets on the other.[298, 299] A diet with a strong restriction of net glucides, sugar and HFCS provides anti-inflammatory and antioxidant lipids such as omega-3 and a few omega-6 that are pro-inflammatory. Among many other health effects, it promotes and restores mitochondrial metabolism.

Omega-6/omega-3 ratio

The *omega-6/omega-3* ratio should be close to or less than 10 and some foods of vegetable origin such as olive oil, nuts and avocados should be part of our usual meals for an optimal diet.

Flax oil, due to its very low index, has specific indications that will be discussed later. (Table 4-2).

Omega-6/omega-3 index.	
Olive oil	13.10
Nuts	5.10
Avocados	13.00
Flax oil	0.24

Table 4-2

Source: own elaboration from Cordani L, *The Paleo Diet*. Ed. John Wiley & Sons, New Jersey 2002

Better omega-3 providers are foods of animal origin present in seafood, fish, fish oil, or the most powerful, krill oil. On the other hand, cod liver oil has been used as a source of vitamins A and D.

A diet such as the one referred to is an anti-inflammatory, anti-angiogenic and pro-apoptotic diet.

The following also protect mitochondrial metabolism: other food-based antioxidants, vitamin C, turmeric, resveratrol, yerba mate, oregano and acyl cysteine and supplements of alpha-lipoic acid, carnitine, coenzyme Q10, magnesium, D ribose and vitamin B complex.

In the ketogenic diet, lipids, which can make up to 70% of the caloric intake, enter the mitochondria directly for energy, but this is limited in cancer cells that do not have metabolic flexibility. Ketone bodies, products of the ketogenic diet, are anti-inflammatory, antioxidant, reduce free radicals and increase the activity of glutathione peroxidase, the essential antioxidant medium of the cell. Ketone bodies also decrease proliferation and angiogenesis in astrocytoma cells.[300-303]

Ketogenic diets with caloric restriction have shown benefits in the treatment of brain cancer, astrocytomas and gliomas, due to anti-inflammatory, anti-angiogenic and pro-apoptosis action. In experimental animals with a ketogenic diet, the direct entry into the mitochondria of acetoacetic acid and butyric acid as an energy source can be seen, avoiding anaerobic glycolysis, which tumour cells are highly dependent on.[304-306]

Omega-3 lipid acids increase apoptosis from mitochondrial metabolism. The increase in apoptosis exerts anti-proliferative and cytotoxic action in tumours.[307-309] Cell proliferation and metastases in cancer are favoured by resistance to apoptosis of the cancer cell, which may be linked to the depletion of mitochondrial metabolism.[268] Damage induced by free radicals by peroxidation of the mitochondrial membrane phospholipids affects permeability, oxidative phosphorylation and DNA structure with mutations and deletions, with severe detriment in energy generation and alterations detected in chronic fatigue syndrome. Lipid replacement therapy together with antioxidants has shown a clear reversal of the syndrome and improvement in neurodegenerative conditions.[310-313]

Omega-3 lipid acids increase apoptosis from mitochondrial metabolism. The increase in apoptosis exerts anti-proliferative and cytotoxic action in tumours.

CHAPTER 5

CEREALS AND PULSES

We have already explained the advantages of vegetables, fruit and meat, which should constitute our usual meals, every day, several times a day.

We have also highlighted the need to avoid sugar and restrict salt.

Table sugar does not exist as such in nature, it is an artificial product derived from the food industry, lacking in nutritional value and only contributes an unnecessary caloric quota and actions that are harmful to health. The craving for sweets can be satisfied, when desired, with moderate consumption, due to the high caloric intake, of honey and dried fruit such as dates, raisins or plums, but must not be confused with candied fruit, which has added sugar.

We also saw that milk and dairy can be consumed, but eventually without being part of our usual meals. They can damage health such as with the risk of unjustifiably supplanting breastfeeding–triggering lactose intolerance, allergy to its various proteins, and undesirable hormonal effects.

Cheese and yoghurt consumed frequently, due to their strong acid loads, induce a calcium-negative balance, with decreased bone density osteopenia and osteoporosis, loss of muscle mass and risk of deterioration in kidney function.

We have also referred to the need to strongly limit the consumption of salt not only at the table but in the kitchen and in the consumption of processed foods that contain it in excess. This is an important means of reducing the risk of cardiovascular disease.

Now we are going to refer to cereals: wheat, oats, barley, rye, rice, corn, millet and sorghum and to pulses: lentils, beans, peas, chickpeas and soya beans.

We do not say goodbye to cereals and pulses. Western cultural, economic and social reality makes it impossible and even more, inconvenient.

If such a statement were to become a reality without due adaptation, which requires gradual changes over time, it would be the cause of a global economic and social crisis.

We can say that as with dairy products, cereals and pulses should not be part of our usual meals, eaten every day several times a day.

Dairy products, *cereals* and *pulses* are not essential; they do not add anything from a nutritional point of view, which meat, fruit and vegetables provide us. They add variety and pleasant tastes, along with proven damages or possible health risks as we are going to consider.

Cereals and pulses as well as pseudocereals such as *quinoa,* chia and buckwheat, cannot be eaten raw, they require prior cooking to inactivate most toxins present. Even several of them, such as quinoa, must be soaked the night before cooking, which gives the water a soapy appearance and must be discarded, in this way part of the toxin is removed but only from the shell, not from its interior.

All the cereals, pseudo-cereals and pulses mentioned are seeds, acidic, with various toxins and some with antinutrients, they can be consumed after cooking and sometimes after soaking, but with limitations, as part of an eventual diet. They do not constitute priority elements for an optimal diet in what should be our usual meals, every day and several times a day, as are fruit, vegetables, meat including fish and other seafood as well as mushrooms.

The seeds of pseudo-cereals and pulses, on the other hand, can be a source of important nutritional contributions through their *sprouts* that contain between 20 and 100 times more nutrients, vitamins, minerals, enzymes and phytochemicals than fully developed plants. Sunflower, lentils, chickpeas, Brussel sprouts, or alfalfa seeds soaked for 10 or 12 hours can be grown at home without pesticides or herbicides. Some can already be harvested after a week and can be kept for a week in the refrigerator.

Cereals, pseudo-cereals and pulses are acidic foods, as are cheeses and yoghurts. Pulses also have antinutrients, which reduce the absorption of important nutrients and the digestion of proteins.

Habitual consumption of these foods produces strong acid loads causing, among other disorders bone demineralization, which makes it necessary to increase the calcium intake. The dairy industry currently adds calcium to milk despite its high calcium content. All this will be duly developed in the respective chapters.

Limitations in the consumption of some of these foods can in certain cases be absolute, a total restriction, such as cereals, especially wheat for coeliacs or broad beans for people with favism. Aside from these cases, the occasional tasting of cheese such as the moderate use of grated cheese in some meals, or for example a plate of cannelloni à la Rossini at an event, some ravioli with chicken and vegetables, or green noodles with pesto, does not interfere with health and they contribute to the gastronomic pleasure and social integration. The limitations with some licenses also fit with regard to alcohol consumption, which due to its importance and significance deserves very special consideration, which will be discussed later on.

Cereals

Coeliac Disease

For those who suffer from the classic form of coeliac disease, the ingestion of even minimal amounts of *gluten* triggers severe autoimmune reactions that damage the intestinal epithelium with pictures of abdominal pain and diarrhoea and the consequent loss of minerals, vitamins, proteins, lipids and glucides. All this configures a malabsorption syndrome that quickly leads to severe malnutrition and systemic inflammation of various organs. In the 1960s it was the most recognized form of coeliac disease. In the 1980s it was recognized that some coeliac disease patients were also diabetic. It has been well documented that some subjects without coeliac disease show gluten sensitivity, which is a determining factor in numerous pathological conditions such as but not limited to, *autism,* depression, migraine, osteoporosis, rheumatic arthritis and irritable bowel syndrome or chronic fatigue.

Coeliac disease occurs in people with greater or lesser susceptibility, which determines the greater or lesser severity of the symptoms and is produced mainly by the undisputed toxicity of gluten *gliadin*, present in wheat flour and also, although to a lesser extent, by prolamines of other cereals: barley and rye and although debatable at present, oats. For these patients, the ingestion of foods with wheat, oats, barley and rye must be totally suppressed.

Coeliac disease manifests itself in various forms: classic, atypical, latent and potential.

The classic form, as we have already mentioned, presents severe intestinal damage, causing profuse diarrhoea with poor absorption of nutrients, malnutrition, oedema, loss of various vitamins and severe dehydration with acidosis.

The atypical form has clinical pictures with few digestive manifestations but with a biopsy-verifiable bowel injury and the presence of anti-gliadin antibodies. Other antibodies, immune complexes, cross-reactivity, and autoantibodies, are causative factors of inflammatory processes due to immune damage to various organs, which causes various diseases, such as proliferative membranous glomerulonephritis[314] or neurological and psychiatric disorders called neurogluten, ataxia, epilepsy, peripheral neuropathy and cognitive disorders such as amnesia, attention deficit with hyperactivity or depression.[315-317]

The latent form does not present clinical manifestations, the intestinal biopsy is normal but there are antigliadin antibodies and autoantibodies, which require periodic controls to detect evolutionary manifestations.[318]

Coeliac disease, gluten sensitivity in non-coeliacs, wheat allergy and irritable bowel can manifest with common symptoms such as diarrhoea, constipation or abdominal pain.

Controls have been carried out on patients with intestinal inflammation syndrome and gluten-free diets since gluten alters intestinal functionalism and gluten-free diets reverted these disorders,[319] among other changes in nutritional elements.[320,321] Coeliac disease disorders are due to an autoimmune reaction triggered by the ingestion of gluten, but autoimmune diseases are produced by the interplay of heredity and environmental factors. The control of these factors is a key point for the treatment of these conditions.[322]

Correcting the increase in intestinal permeability induced by food toxins and improving the integrity of the enterocyte from nutrients derived from fibre by the action of the microbiota are priority resources for the sustainability of the treatment.

Other compounds in addition to gluten may be responsible for intestinal functional and organic damage, such as fructans resulting from glucide fermentation, antinutrient inhibitors of enzymes such as amylase and trypsin, and wheat germ agglutinins and glyphosate.[323,324]

There is genetic conditioning that determines the predisposition or susceptibility to manifest the disease during gluten ingestion which causes mainly intestinal damage but also damages other organs. This damage is of immunological pathogenesis by the presence of *anti-gliadin*, *anti-transglutaminase* and *anti-endomysium* antibodies.

It is interesting to note that human milk induces the maturing of the intestinal immune system in the infant. Lack of breastfeeding determines the introduction of proteins from cow's milk or even soya in children with a family history of diabetes or coeliac disease and increases the production of these diseases. This, together with other observations, has given rise to numerous questions about considering cow's milk as an essential food in the diet.[30]

We mentioned earlier that children for whom the introduction of gluten is carried out while they are still breastfed have 52% fewer incidences of coeliac disease.

The classic form of the disease can be compared to the floating part of an ice floe. Given the non-classical and subclinical forms of the disease,[325] we could say that almost all, or potentially all of us are 'coeliac', or rather we have gluten intolerance.

Gluten means glue; when we mix flour and water the product is the old-fashioned paste, which in the past was used to glue figurines at school but has now been displaced by industrial products.

The old phrase "nobody eats glass" can be changed to "nobody eats paste". The paste must be cooked so that it loses its acute toxicity, this is after adding lipids, be it butter or margarine, salt and sometimes sugar to make it palatable. This dough, baked at high temperatures, by the Maillard reaction glycation of proteins in the crust, generates those delicious flavours, aromas and colours of bread and rolls, often causing addiction.

We have already mentioned that bread has a very high glycemic index, which together with high glucides content means a strong glycemic load. The high glycemic index is given by the fact that 75% of the glucides in wheat are amylopectin A, which is unique in its rapidity to transform into glucose.

A sudden rise in blood glucose with the consequent strong insulin discharge is a situation repeated by the daily diet with bread or other forms of flour, in practically all meals of the day. This eventually leads to insulin resistance, type 2 diabetes, weight gain, obesity, fatty liver, cardiovascular disease and cataracts.

Not only gliadin but other toxins present in cereals, called lectins, increase intestinal permeability, causing the passage of bacterial toxins into the blood, which triggers a cascade of inflammatory reactions that increase the risk of autoimmune diseases, such as rheumatic arthritis,[326] neurodegenerative diseases, including Alzheimer's, and cancer.[327, 329]

Other diseases, including Covid 19, also alter the function of the intestinal barrier due to dysbiosis with the intestinal microbial flora, which aggravates the course of the disease.[330] The *zonulin* protein described in 2000 regulates the permeability of the intestinal and blood-brain barrier through intercellular junctions and by the action of gluten, or a virus that infects and multiplies in the gut, allows autoantibodies to overcome these barriers.[329, 330]

Modern wheat, a product of selection in crops throughout civilization and in the last decades of hybridization, can contain 40 times more gluten than pre-industrial wheat. It has been inferred, although questioned by some, that opioid components of foods with gluten as well as dairy products bind to morphine receptors in the brain, which causes addiction and mild euphoria, which are determinants of stimulation to higher ingestion with an increase of approximately 400 calories per day.

Opioid peptides derived from dietary proteins (exorphins) are found in the urine of patients with autism. A gluten-free and casein-free diet improves autism spectrum symptoms. Five opioid peptides were isolated from wheat gluten. Periodic gastrointestinal upset is common in the general population. Some people with small intakes move the intestine, but most have tolerance and are exposed to autoimmune diseases such as arthritis, fibromyalgia, thyroiditis and neurological disorders such as depression, insomnia, lupus or nephritis. These patients may show positivity for anti-gliadin or anti-transglutaminase antibodies, but it is only these two antibodies that are tested against the many other components of gluten.

Even *autism* has been linked to coeliac disease with or without intestinal manifestation with the common pathogenesis of inflammation triggered by gluten.[331-333] For patients diagnosed as coeliac in any of its forms with gastrointestinal manifestations or only with extra-intestinal manifestations, gluten-free diets for coeliac are encouraged. Gluten-free foods produced by the industry and promoted as essential in the diet of coeliacs are not essential or recommended for coeliacs or non-coeliacs. These foods contain chemical preservatives, soya proteins, industrial seed oils, corn syrup, rice flour, potato starch, tapioca, millet or sorghum, plus added sugar, fructose syrup or sweeteners and are high on the glycemic index and high glycemic load. Gluten-free bread has a glycemic index between 75 and 100. Other gluten-free foods for coeliacs include rice, corn, quinoa, sorghum, flax and amaranth but they are not without adverse health effects due to their content of *lectins* that are also present in wheat, oats, barley and rye. In addition, these foods have up to 90 times more arsenic than the maximum allowed for drinking water. Exposure to arsenic even in low doses leads to headache, fatigue, drowsiness, digestive problems, cardiovascular disease, cancer, respiratory disease and diabetes. Any of the many other components of gluten can cause inflammation and immune responses. All these compounds are natural toxins of the plant with protective action against predators in crops and are strongly active in raw food, which is why foods with wheat flour must be cooked to be edible.

Lectins, in addition to the damage they produce in the intestinal epithelium, which increases permeability producing the so-called punctured intestine, have a harmful action on the peripheral nervous system. This has been observed in experimental studies with rats using histochemical techniques that show the binding of agglutinins in nerve fibres destroying the myelin sheaths. Lectins cross the blood-brain barrier and stimulate the synthesis of inflammatory cytokines.

Although manufactured foods for coeliacs solve the problem of sensitivity to gluten gliadin, they have, as if they were wheat-based, a high glycemic index and high glycemic load, determining strong insulin discharges that over time can generate metabolic syndrome. They are foods of high caloric density and low nutritional value.

Gluten sensitivity is also involved in the production of acne, recurrent stomatitis, vitiligo and atopic dermatitis.

Glyphosate, the most common herbicide used in grain crops and referred to as having minimal toxicity for humans, has been the subject of studies that demonstrate not only its presence in food but also its inhibitory action on enzymatic mechanisms of mammal metabolism.[334] Inhibitory actions on cytochrome P450 enzymes that play an important role in the detoxification of xenobiotics, residual chemical toxins from the environment, have been proven. Synergistically with this, the biosynthesis of aromatic amino acids by bacteria of the intestinal flora is altered.

The referred metabolic interferences, insidiously over time, favour the development of inflammatory processes that intervene in numerous diseases such as gastrointestinal disorders, obesity, diabetes, heart damage, cancer and neurological disorders.

Pulses

In *pulses* in their natural state, the presence of various toxins and antinutrients is recognized. These compounds are mostly inactivated by soaking pulses for six to eight hours and then cooking. Cooking is more effective if done at 130ºC under pressure. The soaking water must be changed prior to cooking. Current biotechnology is working to achieve the total inactivation of these compounds.[335] At present, due to the remaining activity of these products, acute phenomena of discomfort can occasionally be seen after abundant intakes. It cannot be ruled out that minor residual toxicity has pathogenic mediate effects in different organs and tissues, such as those that are listed below.

The nutritional contributions of pulses, due to the lack of sulfur amino acids, methionine and cystine, must be supplemented with cereals, which have them and which in turn, due to the limited content of an essential amino acid lysine, must be supplemented with pulses. Sulfur amino acids are present in meat, eggs and fish.

Among the sulfur amino acids, cystine together with glutamic acid and glycine are glutathione synthesis precursors, the most powerful endogenous antioxidant.

Pulses have alpha galactoside oligosaccharides, raffinose, stachyose and verbascoside that ferment in the intestine and generate short-chain lipid acids responsible for flatulence, which inhibits protein utilization.

Phytates in pulses as well as in cereals can form insoluble chelates making the absorption of calcium, magnesium, zinc, iron and copper difficult and also making it difficult to digest proteins. As some of these proteins are vitamin transporters, pictures of vitaminic deficiencies can be presented. Poor protein digestion and absorption also hinder glutathione synthesis.

Among the toxins we have:

Lectins

These are glycoproteins that adhere to glucides in the intestinal wall of the duodenum and jejunum and cause cellular damage by increasing intestinal permeability, which allows their passage into the blood along with bacteria and toxins. This has led to the so-called leaky gut syndrome. Altered intestinal permeability is associated with pathologies such as Crohn's disease, atopic eczema, chronic giardiasis, intestinal candidiasis or coeliac disease. It can also trigger infections and allergies, and anti-lectin antibodies in IgA, IgG, IgM and IgE with cross-reactivity to various tissue antigens, contributing to the pathogenesis of autoimmune diseases such as arthritis.[336]

It has been observed that lectins block the response to leptins in hypothalamic centres, which are hormones secreted by adipocytes in fatty tissue, their concentration in serum is proportional to the amount of fatty tissue. Leptin on receptors located in the hypothalamus has a double action: it decreases appetite and, like thyroxine, stimulates metabolism producing greater energy expenditure. The blockade of hypothalamic leptin receptors would be a contributing factor to weight gain and obesity.[337]

Other toxins

Saponins

Although their toxicity is scarce by the oral route, some effects described by these compounds have been hemolysis and intestinal alterations.

Lathyrogens

Continuous and abundant intake of pulses, such as grass pea (Lathirussatirus) or peas commonly consumed in periods of hunger in Central India, due to neurotoxic compounds, can cause serious neurological problems, and disorders called *neurolathyrism*.

Divicin and convincine

A genetic disease linked to chromosome X is the deficiency of the enzyme glucose-6-phosphate dehydrogenase which is the most common enzyme deficiency in the world. This reduces the antioxidant potency of haemoglobin by reducing NAD, the cause of haemolytic anaemia after ingestion of vicine and convicine, powerful oxidants contained in fava beans, in a disease called *fabism.*

Antinutrients, Phytates

They produce insoluble chelates by binding to minerals which makes their absorption difficult and also affects protein digestibility.

The presence of *antinutrient* compounds makes it essential to cook pulses, by which most of them are inactivated, but biotechnology is still working to achieve the total elimination of these compounds.

There is no nutritional contribution of cereals or pulses that is not supplied by meat, fruit and vegetables. Both cereals and pulses can be ingested only occasionally and should not be included in regular meals.

CHAPTER 6

EVOLUTION

Where do we come from and where are we going?

To effectively integrate the knowledge of the anatomical and physiological characteristics of our body in eating behaviour, it is necessary to know our *evolution*, and where we come from in order to understand where we are and where we are going. Photo 6-1

The human species has been in existence for two million years, or somewhat more, with an evolutionary process of six or seven million years from the hominids that preceded the proper bipeds, the hominins.

Two or seven million years would seem like a long process, but it is not if we compare it with the 160 million years that the dinosaurs lasted, which became extinct 65 million years ago.

It has been calculated that reducing the entire history of the earth to one year, starting from zero hours on 1 January, *Homo sapiens sapiens* appears in the last four minutes of 31 December.

Until now, the human species has been very successful if we consider its extension throughout the planet and the increase for the individual in life expectancy, but in biology, extinction is not the exception but the rule.

Our history is so recent that it would seem impossible to predict what our future will be, but evolution up to the present has been plotted.

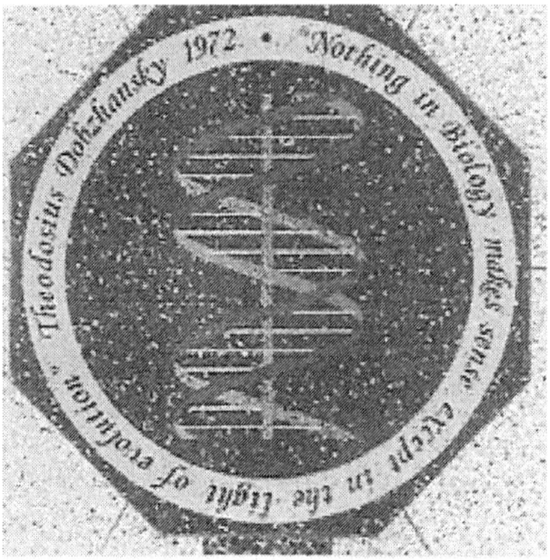

"Nothing in biology makes sense except in the light of evolution"
—Theodosius Dobzhansky

Photo 6-1: Medallion mosaic on the floor of the Jordan Hall of Science. University of Notre Dame

Our ancestors

The first of our ancestors were the pre-australopithecines, with four species of which *Ardipithecus Ramidusa* (belonging to Ardi), from four to six million years ago and *Australopithecus afarensis* (to which Lucy belongs) from three to four million years ago. Both Ardi and Lucy's remains were found in northeast Africa, in Ethiopia, in 1994 and 1974 respectively. More recently, in 2008 in South Africa the remains of another species were found, the *Autralopithecussediba*, from two million years ago; possibly a collateral branch without being a direct ancestor of the genus *Homo*.

These ancestors are followed by the genus Homo: *Homo habilis, Homo ergaster* or the African Homo *erectus* (Java man and Peking man), *Homo sapiens* (Neardental and Denisovan) and *Homo sapiens sapiens* (*Cro-magnon* and modern man).

Based on paleoanthropology by means of chemical analysis of coprolites and the content of carbon, nitrogen (isotopes N_{14} / N_{15}), erbium and zinc in bone fossils and marks or deterioration of the teeth, it is deduced that the meals of Australopithecines were based on vegetables, nuts, insects and small mammals.

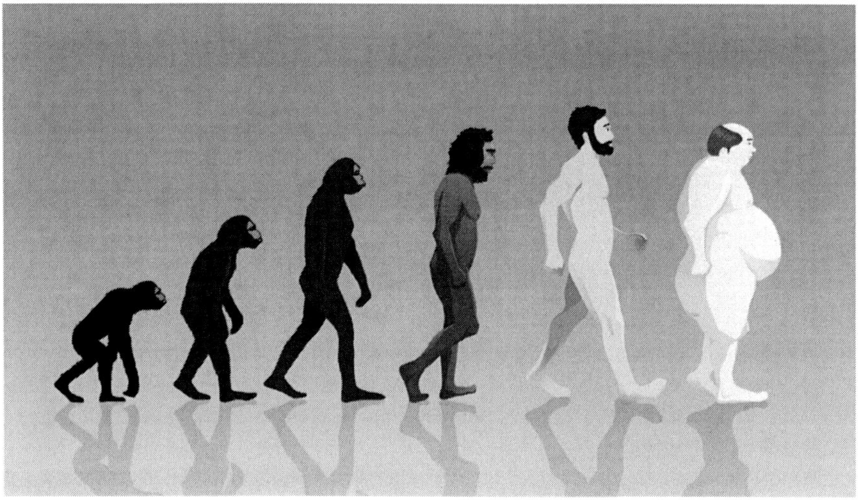

Fig. 6-1: Human evolution

The *Homo habilis* of two million years ago knew how to use fire but did not produce it and ate vegetables and fruit and occasionally meat, especially bone marrow, breaking the bones left by scavengers, with stones.

The *Homo erectus* of 1.5 million years ago lasted more than 10 times as long as the modern human being, homo sapiens sapiens and was the first to leave Africa; remains were found as the Java Man of 700 thousand years ago, the Peking Man from 400 thousand years ago and *Homo antecessor* from 1 million years ago in Europe, Spain and Italy.[338]

Homo ergaster remained in Africa. They are who developed a more elaborate way of stone carving called Achelense or Mode 2; perhaps this allowed them to displace those who followed the old technique (Olduvayense) who had to emigrate from Africa.

Homo sapiens such as the *Neanderthal*, whose remains were found in the Neander Valley in Germany and lived from 250,000 to 50,000 years ago, and the Denisovan, whose remains were identified in Siberia and lived from 400,000 to 50,000 years ago, lived during the last glaciation adapting to it in caves or homes dug underground, keeping bonfires lit. They were hunters and specialized in hunting large arctic mammals such as mammoths and hairy rhinoceros. They covered themselves with furs and buried their dead. They were predominantly carnivores, the men consuming 5,000 calories per day and the women 4,000 due to the high energy expenditure of the physical rigour of their lives in the prevailing low temperatures.

Neanderthals were displaced by modern humans, *sapiens sapiens*, to disappear on the periphery of their range (the Iberian Peninsula, the Rock of Gibraltar, the high plateaus of Croatia and the vicinity of the Arctic Circle) between 28,000 and 35,000 years ago.

Homo sapiens sapiens, modern humans, according to some, migrated from Africa 90 or 60 thousand years ago. They advanced north, east and west as the ice retreated. They arrived in Australia on rustic rafts 25 thousand years ago, others say 70 thousand years ago and crossed the Bering Strait, which was not yet covered by water, 30 thousand years ago to descend to America, reaching Tierra del Fuego 10,000 years ago.

They spread and populated almost the entire planet across five continents (Antarctica was discovered by the Spanish Gabriel de Castilla in 1603 and began to be populated in 1904).

Europe only just began to be populated by modern man, sapiens sapiens, some 40 thousand years ago, since it is assumed that the Syrian desert was an insurmountable barrier for millennia between Africa and Europe.

A prehistoric group from 32 thousand years ago is the Cro-Magnon man who, like the Neanderthal, lived through the last ice age and had the same cranial capacity that was greater than that of *Homo erectus*. From the Cro-Magnons the first artists emerged.

The evolutionary process up to the present did not follow a linear model, but a candlestick model; it was made up of ramifications in various species, which at various times coexisted and then became extinct except for Homo sapiens sapiens. However, genetic studies show that there were crossovers; in the genome of Europeans there are between 1 and 4% of Neanderthal genes,[339] and in the genome of south-eastern New Guinea inhabitants there have 3% Davisonian genes.[340,341]

In the evolution toward standing upright, the foramen magnum, where the vertebral column is inserted, moves from the back of the skull forward, almost to the middle of the skull. The spine becomes almost rectilinear moving almost 90 degrees on the pelvis, which widens. With the acquisition of a standing gait, running speed decreases and longer walks are possible with less sun exposure. With the widening of the pelvis, the greater cranial development and the greater length and sinuosity of the birth canal, although they allow the vaginal delivery of foetuses with larger skulls, the births were mostly difficult and premature.

The thumb of the foot in apes is transverse with the ability to grasp. In humans, the thumb of the foot is parallel to the other toes, allowing balance and forward momentum in gait.

Standing upright allows, in addition to releasing the upper limbs, scanning the horizon and avoiding overheating through the breeze. The arms are released whilst marching.

In mammals, the larynx is high, allowing simultaneous breathing and swallowing. In humans, the larynx opens at the oropharynx. Breathing and swallowing alternate, but the larynx makes clearer and more diverse sounds than language allows. At birth, the larynx has not descended and hence choanal atresia is incompatible with life, the baby cannot breathe through the mouth and becomes cyanised, cries and at that moment the larynx lowers and allows some air to enter. In addition to the greater brain development, there is the greater development of the cortex, which means that the brain requires 20% of the body's energy.

The neonate chimpanzee has 65% of the brain capacity of the adult, and humans have 25% of the capacity that they acquire at 45 years, which is when the brain fully develops.

The continuous growth of the brain in the development of our species, the encephalization process, was carried out as a consequence of standing upright and the food transition from vegetarianism to omnivorism, with the incorporation of meat as an important protein source.

This change in diet, which meant the passage of Australopithecus vegetarianism to Homo erectus omnivorism, led to a shortening of the intestine and the time devoted to meals. This, together with the release of the upper limbs and standing upright, led to progressive encephalization.

Food transitions[342]

The provision of proteins from exclusively vegetables is evident in the growth and development of sheep, cattle and horses whose natural and healthiest food is through grazing. However, this takes long hours for the large intake necessary to cover the protein requirement and also a large digestive system.

The breakdown of cellulose, hemicellulose and pectin membranes that surround the plant cells, which despite containing 90% water give them body, is not carried out by enzymes but by the intestinal bacterial flora in a long fermentation process in the various gastric cavities through which the food passes after regurgitation, which is rumination.

Bipedalism and encephalization

In the human species, the erect position and the gait on the lower limbs, bipedalism, developed together with the food transition that incorporated meat as an important protein source, which reduced the volume of the digestive system and the necessary hours dedicated to meals. Digestion of animal proteins is carried out easily and in a short time due to the action of the high acidity of gastric juices with a pH of 1. With bipedalism, the upper limbs are released, and the hips widen. Together with this, cranial capacity progressively increases with greater growth and development of the brain, a process called *encephalization*.

Carnivores or herbivores? What are the anatomical and functional characteristics of our body that condition it to eat what kinds of foods?

The anatomical and physiological characteristics of our body show us that we are not conditioned to eat food exclusively from the plant kingdom or exclusively from the animal kingdom. Herbivorous animals must consume large amounts of vegetables to meet their protein requirement. This requires a long digestive system and a long residence time for food to carry out its digestion.

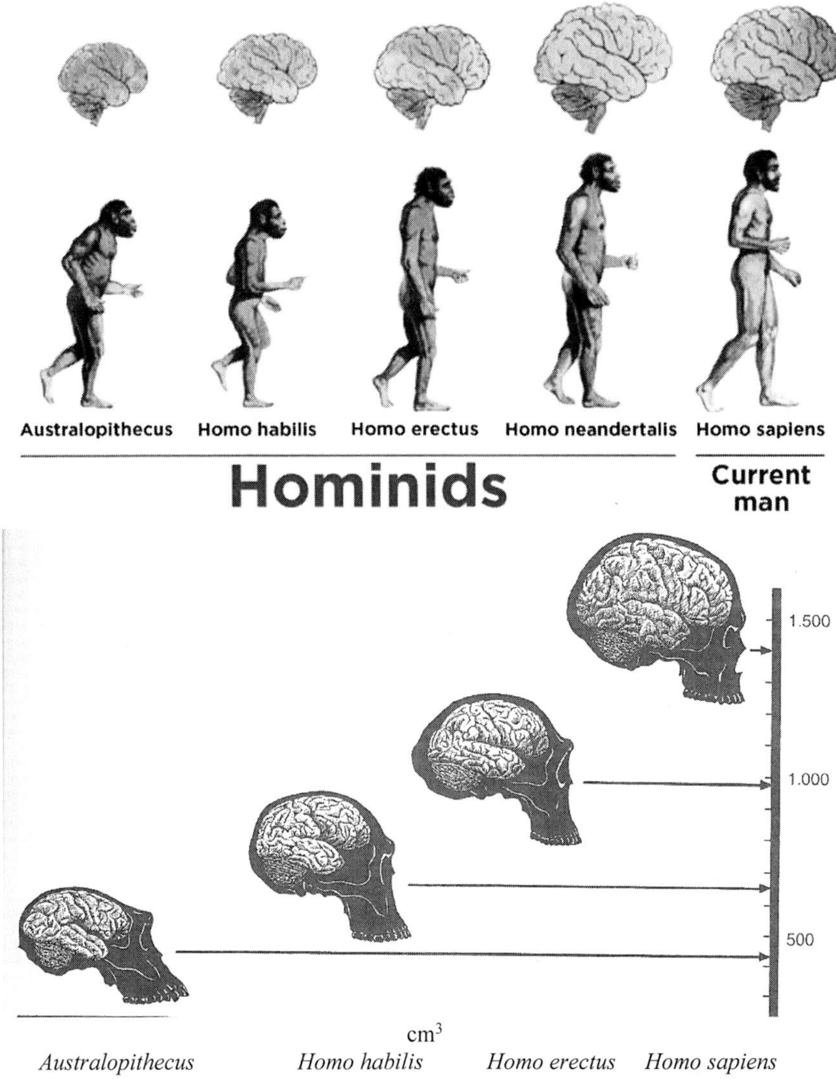

Fig. 6-2: Encephalization

Anatomy of the digestive system

Herbivores, Carnivores, Omnivores

Vegetables have a cell wall made up of cellulose, hemicellulose and pectin digested by bacterial flora in a prolonged fermentation process. If we take as an example a bovine, a typical *herbivorous* animal, we can see that it has a stomach with four cavities through which the food passes after being regurgitated.

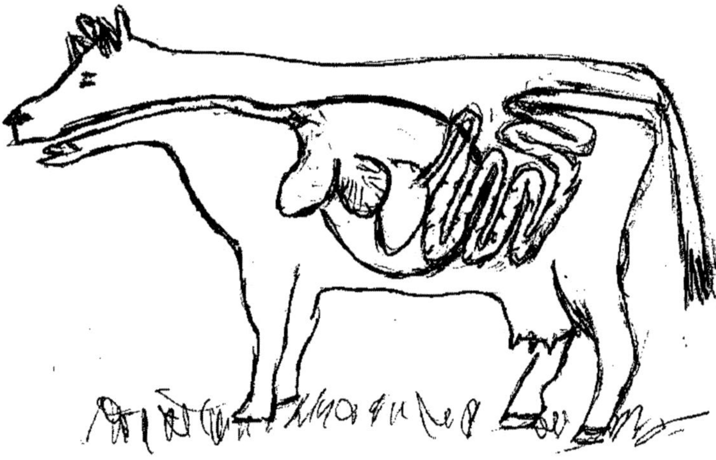

Fig. 6-3: Anatomy of the digestive system of the cow

The anatomy of a *carnivore* is very different, it has a much simpler and shorter digestive system, as we can see taking the wolf as an example.

This is because the meat is digested by stomach acidity with a pH of 1 and requires much less time.

A herbivore has flat teeth and the jaw movement is up and down vertically and right and left laterally. This is appropriate to fulfil a shredding function.

A carnivore has sharp, pointed teeth and prominent canines. The lower incisors in the bite are located behind the upper denture in a scissor motion. The lower jaw is displaced anteroposteriorly, suitable to bite the prey and cut the meat.

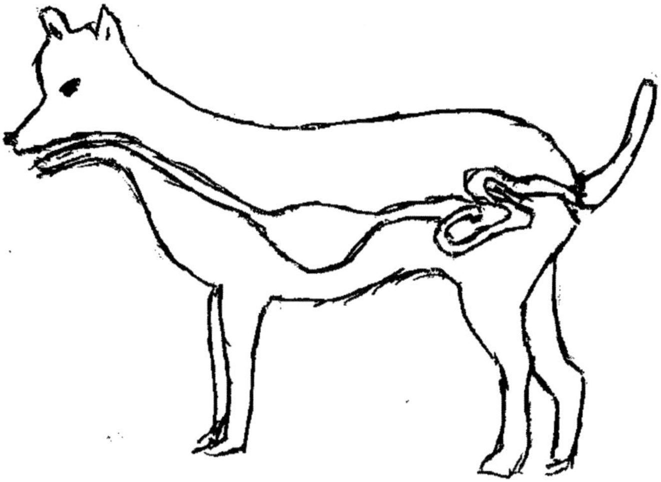

Fig. 6-4: Anatomy of the digestive system of the wolf

As *omnivores,* we have flat molars and premolars suitable for grinding like herbivores, sharp incisors and canines for biting, in which the lower incisors slide behind the upper incisors as in carnivores, in a scissor motion suitable for cutting meat. The lower jaw moves vertically, anteroposteriorly and laterally, combining what is observed in herbivores and carnivores. Saliva has the enzyme, amylase, like herbivores, to initiate glucides digestion.

Starch stability has allowed palaeontology to contribute interesting information about our ancestors' diet.

Homo sapiens have three times more amylase in the pancreas and salivary glands than chimpanzees, which helps survival during times of lack of meat and fruit. This occurred two million years ago and is associated with high brain development.

Conditioning of our species as omnivores is evident not only by shorter intestine length but by lower gastric capacity compared to a vegetarian animal. Cattle have a stomach with four cavities with a volume between

120 and 200 litres, while in humans the stomach has a capacity of 1 to 1.5 litres, 150 times less.

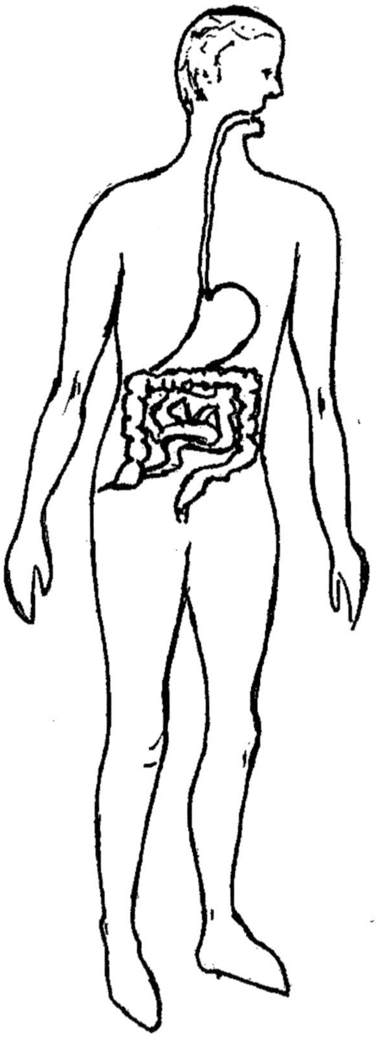

Fig. 6-5: Anatomy of the digestive system of a human.

We are not conditioned to be exclusively vegetarian like cattle or sheep or exclusively carnivorous like cats.

The human organism is conditioned to ingest food from the animal and vegetable kingdoms and that means omnivore. But the term omnivore does not mean, as it could be interpreted literally, that it can eat everything or anything. You cannot eat everything, there are natural or industrial products that are toxic, with acute, chronic, manifest or latent toxicity or without being properly toxic, but produce an intolerance.

CHAPTER 7

OPTIMAL MEALS

"De humani corporis fabrica" said Andrés Vesalio, Professor of Anatomy in Padua in the middle of the 16th century, considered to be the father of anatomy.

The human body can be seen as a machine, so complex and sophisticated that, as Vesalius said, it is a factory, it generates various products, even other machines.

The human body, like all living beings, does not need a central command or even an operator to start it up, it is autonomous and has multiple and versatile functions, such as growth, reproduction, maintenance, repair and like all animals, locomotion. In addition, like higher animals, it has complex brain functions, which reach the consciousness of transcendence. To fulfil these tasks, the contribution of plastic materials and energy sources is necessary.

As the plastic materials, we highlight proteins in the first place. As an energy source, glucides and lipids, fuels that when burned through chemical reactions as part of metabolism, release energy.

If the necessary proteins are not provided, the growth, maintenance and repair of cells grouped in tissues, which make up the structure of the various organs, which are the pieces of this complex machinery, are limited to a variable degree.

If glucides and lipids are not provided, energy is obtained by burning proteins, which we call protein catabolism, which subtracts proteins for cell growth and repair. In addition, residual acid ash from protein catabolism increases, which tends to produce acidosis. Acidosis is inconvenient for the body because, among other harmful effects, it causes the loss of calcium with demineralization and decreases bone mass to a slight degree, osteopenia or to a marked degree, osteoporosis facilitating the production of fractures.

As plastic foods, since they are also part of the composition of tissues, in addition to proteins we have 17 minerals: chlorine, sodium, potassium, calcium, phosphorus, magnesium and in small quantities, called microelements, copper, cobalt, chromium, manganese, zinc, fluorine, iron, molybdenum, selenium, aluminium and iodine.

Not only plastic and energy foods are necessary for nutrition, but there is also a third type of food, the thirteen vitamins that act as catalysts or activators of the chemical reactions that make the cellular metabolism. Without vitamins, food cannot normally fulfil its nutritional role. The great teacher of nutrition, Pedro Escudero said:

> To produce an explosion, the existence of gunpowder is not enough, it is essential that the fulminant or prime acts...and just as the same fulminant or prime does not serve indistinctly for any explosive, the functions of nutrition also require different vitamins depending on the type of food used[343]

Pedro Escudero, during the First World War in 1914, stimulated the study of nutrition, which until then, because it was something so common, had been of little scientific interest. In the USA, Great Britain and Japan, scientific research departments have been created for studies on food, such as in Japan, the Imperial Institute of Nutrition in Tokyo, in Russia the Scientific Institute of Nutrition in Odesa and then others in Moscow, Leningrad and Kyiv. Specialized publications and reviews studying scientific, industrial and economic aspects of food, seeking to adapt the diet to the population according to their needs and schools for the training of nutritionists and dietitians arise. Escudero was the pioneer with a big transcendence in Latin American countries. This author met Ramos Galván in the children's hospital in Mexico in 1969 when he went from the United States for joint research on nutrition and he was told by Professor Ramos Galván with great pride that he had studied nutrition in Buenos Aires with Pedro Escudero.

The book *Alimetación* dedicated to the education of the population presents the lectures at the headquarters of the newspaper *La Prensa*. In that book, Escudero says that the body is like a machine that needs fuel, lipids and glucides, protein for repairs and vitamins for bodily processes. He refers to deficiency diseases, avitaminosis and autophagy until death from starvation when it loses 33% of its theoretical weight. Also, the author refers to the quality, quantity and proportion of nutrients, and the minerals, calcium, phosphorus, sodium and potassium.

He highlights the value of meat with viscera, especially liver, kidney, snails, brains, and tripe and noted that more than 33% of protein calories are toxic.

Also in 1933 Escudero distinguished between acidic and alkaline foods and recommended the suspension of all acidic foods 48 hours before a sports competition. Below we transcribe some of the paragraphs:

> Food can be acidic or alkaline, also called basic. The degree of reaction is not measured at the time of ingestion but in the ashes that remain after their complete use in the body. *Eating* acidic foods favours the appearance of acidosis…; eating alkaline foods avoids or neutralizes it. Acidosis is easy to achieve from fasting, exercise and die

Referring to sports competitions he said:

> Forty-eight hours before the final test, the athlete will prepare morally and materially…. His diet will be preferably alkaline; he will suppress all meat, even white ones….He will cut out bread, eggs and all grains

Unfortunately, this was later relegated to oblivion until the subject was taken up again with all the interest and significance it deserves.

Vitamins come from food, they are essential because they cannot be synthesized by the human organism, with the exception of vitamin D, synthesized in the skin by the action of solar radiation and later transformed into more active forms in the liver and kidney, and vitamin K, synthesized in the intestine by the bacterial flora.

Not only is the contribution of materials necessary, mainly proteins and minerals, vitamins and energy through glucides and lipids, but the quality of food is especially important. Returning to the didactic expositions of the master Escudero, we transcribe the following paragraph:

> The organism is a federation of organs, the organs a society of tissues, the tissues a harmonious grouping of cells. The cell is an unstable chemical system, of variable composition and at the mercy of the quality and quantity of the food that is ingested. Insufficient or inadequate meals modifies the structure and size of the organs[344].

The quality of the inputs must be that for which the machine has been designed.

If a mechanical transport vehicle has been designed to operate with gasoline and we put diesel, kerosene, alcohol or gas in, it may not work or do so with less or minimum performance and suffer deterioration that can lead to its destruction.

The contribution in quantity, proportion or quality or inadequate nutrients gives rise to very diverse diseases.

For diseases arising due to an insufficient quantity of nutrients, globally referred to as deficiency diseases, we have protein malnutrition and protein-calorie malnutrition, vitamin deficiencies, called avitaminosis, mineral deficiencies such as bone demineralization or iron deficiency anaemia, or thyroid insufficiency due to lack of iodine. Diseases due to excessive amounts of nutrients are mainly due to excessive caloric intake that leads to weight gain, obesity and various consequent diseases. If to this we add inadequate proportion and quality of nutrients, we have a wide range of very diverse diseases that can occur directly or indirectly as a consequence of food. To the old saying: "tell me who you are with, and I will tell you who you are", we can add: "tell me what you eat and I will tell you how you are going".

This gives reason to that old medical adage that there are no diseases but sick people. On the other hand, with optimal meals, a state of health can be achieved, without major differences between one person and another. With an adequate lifestyle that avoids a sedentary lifestyle and follows optimal meals, the achievement and maintenance of health are highly feasible.

In an anecdotal concept, relative and limited to the purely organic, we can say that health is the silence of the organs, but health is more than that, it is not only the absence of disease. As defined by the WHO, health is the state of complete physical, mental and social well-being. This implies the balance of the individual with the natural and social environment in which they live.

In the following topics we will develop:

1) The optimal quality of meals for the human body.
2) How to avoid a sedentary lifestyle, with the greatest benefits and the least risks.
3) The balance between the natural and social environment, which implies ethical-moral development.

Plastic and energetic elements necessary for our body are provided by food, just as our automobile fuel, lubricants and necessary spare parts are provided by service stations and garages.

For our car, we do not need to know the structure of the engine or how it works to acquire and supply the appropriate class of inputs. This is known by the manufacturer, specified in the manual with which it leaves the factory and is carried out by garage mechanics.

For our body, we need to know its structure and its function, since we are the ones who provide its inputs through our food, and we do not come into the world with a manual.

It is different with animals due to genetic inheritance encoded in DNA as their behaviour is guided by instinct and parental imitation if they live in their natural environment. The human being has largely and increasingly withdrawn from nature, currently in an alarming way. We have already seen that in the development of human beings not only genetic inheritance but also social inheritance, that is, the cultural acts, which come first from the family (and from very early mainly by the primary caregiver), then by a school, a club and other institutions. In this aspect, mass media, mainly television and increasingly the Internet, acquire a relevant role.

Culture acts in a wide variety of ways, repressing, modifying, conditioning or altering instinctual behaviours with positive, negative or unpredictable effects according to interests or values.

For our species, a high degree of developed consciousness is not the only priority but also the quality of life that we can have.

The lifestyles typical of different cultures, addictions, physical activity and habitual diet are essential aspects to be considered as determinants of the state of health or disease of individuals and society.

Food and nutrition, for several years, have been a matter of concern for medical societies but not in the full dimension they deserve, neither with the adequate support of government powers nor with the necessary autonomy outside of marketing by food-producing companies.

It is a priority to promote together with lifestyle habits, eating behaviours from childhood and agreement between medical associations, government powers, non-governmental organizations such as consumer protection, organizations and industrial companies and the production, marketing and advertising campaigns of food.

Natural, processed and ultra-processed foods

We can consider foods in three groups.

Group 1: natural, unprocessed or minimally processed foods. **Group 2:** processed foods. **Group 3:** ultra-processed foods.[345,346]

Group 1

Natural foods, unprocessed or minimally processed foods

We can recognize parts of plants, animals or fungi, such as leafy vegetables, roots, tubers, fruit, meat, poultry, fish, eggs or honey. They can be in the natural state or minimally processed, such as dried, crushed, chilled, frozen, boiled or vacuum packed. No added sugar, sweeteners, salt or any other additive except for spices.

Group 2

Processed foods

Foods of the previous group are recognized, but with processing that seeks greater durability or improves sensory conditions that make them especially palatable. For this, sugar, salt, vegetable oils (from seeds) industrial kinds of vinegar and up to four other additives are added. Cooked at a high temperature in the oven, grilled or fried with the consequent changes in colour, aroma and flavour typical of glycation.

Group 3

Ultra-processed foods

Natural foods are not recognized or only as a small part. They have added sugar or sweeteners, salt and more than five various ingredients such as colourants, flavourings, emulsifiers, humectants or anti-caking agents. They include ultra-processed foods such as pizzas, cakes, packaged desserts, hamburgers, sausages, sugary drinks with various additives, energy drinks, some kinds of pasta, snacks, cereal bars, yoghurts, ready-to-eat products, smoked meat, powders for soups, artisan cheeses, fish, canned goods, infant formulas, industrial bread, biscuits and cakes.

Processed and ultra-processed foods are foods low in fibre, vitamins and minerals, with high caloric density. Regular consumption is a determinant of weight gain, obesity, high blood pressure, cardiovascular disease, cancer, insulin resistance and diabetes. This is already endemic in many countries: weight gain, obesity, type 2 diabetes, hypertension, metabolic syndrome and demineralization; pathologies that are on the rise indicate the failure of various recommended diets.

Bisphenol and *phthalates* are products incorporated in the internal coatings of plastic containers for many ultra-processed foods and studies of the concentration of these products in urine show a contributing relationship in the pathogenesis of the chronic diseases referred to. These products act as endocrine disruptors favouring the development of insulin resistance, diabetes, cardiovascular disease, weight gain and obesity.[347,348]

The aforementioned consequence of technological advances and economic interests presents us with the challenge of maintaining or restoring a dynamic balance between control and adaptation in the face of changes. The answers to this challenge will give the level of health or disease and even life expectancy of current and future generations.

The strong development of this theme in undergraduate and graduate teaching programmes and its dissemination in the general population will contribute to achieving an evidence-based diet, taking away space from a diet based on market interests. This concept has been referred to in a broader context, referring to medicine as a whole.[349]

The economy is today the most powerful engine that moves society, but evidence-based medicine and food are part of medicine, and the medical profession must act on government powers, non-governmental organizations and industrial companies to set the course that must be given to that engine to achieve health in its broadest sense, which means the well-being of the entire population. The ambitious slogan "Health for all in the year 2000" that was announced at the International Conference on Primary Health Care, Alma-Ata, Kazakhstan (a province of the then USSR in 1978), organized by WHO, PAHO (the Pan American Health Organization) and Unicef, today seems like a chimaera.

Acidic and alkaline foods

There are foods that when metabolize, generate alkaline residues while other foods generate acid residues (*alkaline and acidic foods*). Sources of acids in food are meat, cereals, pulses and dairy products: cheeses and yoghurts.

Mainly in Western industrialized countries, 50% of the acid production is given by sulfates derived from the oxidation of sulfur amino acids and the rest by phosphates derived from the hydrolysis of phosphoproteins and phospholipids. Also, due to the excessive use of salt in the diet as sodium chloride, which is an acidifying salt. These acids are first neutralized by the bicarbonate of the plasma as well as being excreted by the kidney, directly acidifying the urine and producing ammonia. Ammonia production is made from muscle-derived glutamine.

The need to reconsider values as the normal reference of the equilibrium state between acidity and alkalinity of the blood (pH and CO_3H^-)has been postulated, that is where *net acid excretion* (NAE) = zero.[350] With persistently high acid excretion, there is a mobilization of buffers from bone tissue with consequent demineralization and a state defined as mild metabolic acidosis. With a diet based mainly on cereals, especially rice and wheat, pulses, and foods of animal origin, (meat and dairy derivatives such as cheese and yoghurts) there is an increased generation of acids and a decreased availability of alkalis for their neutralization. In this type of diet, the use of vinegar, which is acetic acid, also contributes to the acid load. Apple cider vinegar, which is already acetic acid, if not purified, (i.e. virgin apple cider vinegar produced at home), leaves alkaline residues when it metabolizes. Shop-bought ones are acidic, like any other vinegar and they look transparent because of purification.

This determines that organic liquids tend to increase their concentration of acids and decrease their concentration of alkalines. In the diet, the acidic foods referred to, of which meat should not be lacking in an optimal diet, should be neutralized with two or three servings of fruit and vegetables.

A mixed salad of fruit and vegetables begins its *digestion* during chewing due to the action of ptyalin in the mouth and after swallowing the food, the bolus passes quickly to the intestine where digestion is completed in the alkaline medium. After this, meat can be ingested and digested in the stomach in an acid medium with hydrochloric acid with the closure of the pylorus. If fruit and vegetables are ingested together with meat or immediately after, they are trapped in the stomach by the closure of the pylorus and they ferment giving gastric distention by flatulence, favouring gastroesophageal reflux, esophagitis and even diaphragmatic hernia.

Gastroesophageal reflux with long-standing oesophagitis with increased severity predisposes to the transformation of oesophagal epithelium, termed Barrett's oesophagus, a precursor of oesophagal carcinoma.

If we add virgin apple vinegar to the meat when it is eaten, this neutralizes the acidity of the meat. Likewise, salting of the meat should be done not only with kitchen salt, which is sodium chloride but also with a mixture of two parts of sodium chloride and one part of sodium bicarbonate. Sodium chloride is acidifying and the mixture with sodium bicarbonate in the physiological proportion referred to is better.

In an acidic diet such as referred to with cereals, pulses, meat, cheeses and yoghurts, with low consumption of fruit and vegetables, the body responds first to neutralize excess acids mainly through plasma bicarbonate, whose availability is limited by the least contribution of precursors in the diet. Consequently, acid accumulation has a significant impact on bone and kidneys.

Bone is an important alkaline reservoir, mainly calcium and potassium carbonate and phosphate, which is mobilized by the effect of acidosis, causing a loss of bone mass and osteopenia over time. The kidneys increase acid elimination and ammonia synthesis (urinary acidification and ammonia genesis). By acidifying the urine, a new synthesis of bicarbonate is produced restoring blood bicarbonate, but the calcium from the bones is lost through urine. Acidosis over time also determines the loss of muscle mass, and sarcopenia, due to glutamine release used by the kidney for ammonia synthesis.

With a strong acid load resulting from intense exercise, infection or an acidic diet from eating meat, cereals and pulses, cheeses and yoghurt and very little consumption of fruit and vegetables, blood bicarbonate and urine acidification are not enough to maintain the acid-base balance of the blood. In this situation, calcium carbonate is mobilized from the bones and renal ammonia genesis occurs with ammonium excretion, which increases acid excretion, that is, the hydrogen ion.

Ammonium excretion is of a special category, different to excretion of other elements such as urea or phosphates that are eliminated to a greater or lesser extent to regulate the concentration in the blood and increases when glomerular filtration decreases but only up to a certain limit. It is a regulation with limitation, a limitation that occurs when decreasing the glomerular filtration rate to 25%. Ammonium excretion is carried out at maximum capacity and as an eventual measure in face of a strong acid load, the capacity does not increase with a decrease in glomerular filtration rate that normally occurs at an advanced age.[351] With an acid diet, if it is usual, the permanent activity of the kidney in ammonio genesis could be the factor that favours renal sclerosis. The consequent effect of *acidosis* could be osteopenia, sarcopenia and nephrosclerosis.

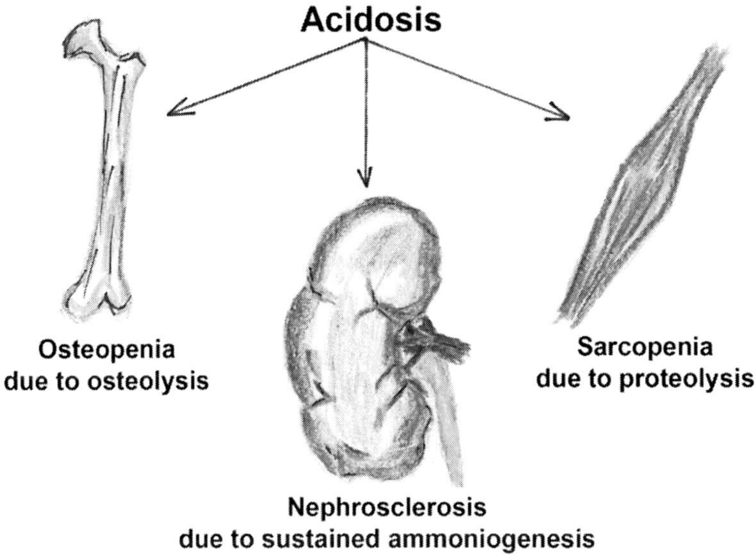

Fig. 7-1: Effect of acidosis on the skeletal, muscular and renal structure
Source: Voyer, Luis E. Medio interno. "Fisiología, patología y tratamiento de los líquidos orgánicos". Ed. Journal. Buenos Aires. 2017: 89 - 90.

It should be noted that 25% of adults with chronic kidney failure that leads to hemodialysis or transplantation have no prior history of kidney or urological diseases. In these patients, chronic kidney failure is discovered by analysis during health check-ups. The decline in renal function with age makes it even more difficult to eliminate acid residues generated by diet and consequent disorders increase. Differences have been shown in blood and urine acidity indicators according to age from youth to old age and in populations with different eating habits. It is observed that in the elderly the effect of a high acid load is increased by diet. Among these effects, people over 50 years of age show a higher incidence of hip fracture, but not so in populations in which the diet provides abundant precursors of alkaline residues.

Virgin apple vinegar is not purified and has a cloudy appearance. Despite containing acetic acid like all vinegar, as a product of aerobic fermentation, when metabolized in the body it leaves alkaline residual products. Used daily in food, especially with salad, even with meat, it is a contributing factor to an alkaline diet that maintains the pH and blood bicarbonate in optimal values. It can also be ingested daily in dilution of one or two teaspoons in a glass of water. This has also been declared beneficial in the prevention of staphylococcal furunculosis and by local application for the vitality of skin and hair.

Virgin apple cider vinegar can be made at home as described in the final chapter. The one that is bought in shops is acidic and crystalline because it is purified.

Functional Foods

The concept of *functional foods* was proposed in 1980 in Japan and quickly spread to Europe, America and practically all cities, especially in the developed world. In these regions, the alarming increase in chronic diseases such as obesity, diabetes, hypertension, cardiovascular disease, stroke and cancer,[352] to which we must add osteoporosis, neurodegenerative diseases and kidney failure, constitute an endemic and global problem. If this situation is not reversed, the growing social cost due to absenteeism or work limitation and the permanent increase in the budget for medical care will occur, together with an ever greater deterioration in the quality of life. Likewise, it can already be foreseen that the increase in life expectancy at birth that we have been observing as a consequence of the decrease in infant mortality and control of infectious diseases, may already present a plateau or even decrease due to mortality resulting from the referred to diseases. There is no other way to reverse this situation, although not immediately, than the education of consumers, producers and governing powers.

Science with a conscience: science, technology and industry in themselves do not have ethics, but those who fulfil the development of science, technology and industry and all society members who use the contributions of science, technology and industry, must do so within an ethical framework.

There is a preference for hypercaloric processed foods due to the addition of bad fats such as margarine and bad glucides such as sugar or fructose syrup replacing fresh foods such as fruit and vegetables. Add to this an excessive consumption of salt and a sedentary lifestyle.

At the Second Food Summit Ministry of Health, Buenos Aires 2015, Argentina was referred to as the world's leading country in the consumption of bread, soft drinks and sodium.

Education must enable every individual in the family and in society to be a zealous guardian of health.

In scientific, technological and industrial companies, there should be no interest that subordinates avoiding harm, promoting the good of users and preserving the environment.

Those who exercise governmental power must take into account that politics is to act within an ethical framework, and it is necessary to educate the leaders who represent the people as this has a cascading effect on future generations because producers and rulers come from the people.

While this long process, like any educational process, is being carried out, the development of biotechnology in the food industry with incipient but growing legislation in this regard motivates the population in the search for alternative measures, with an increasing supply of special food products; functional foods.

The concept of functional foods is a bit elastic and can be considered debatable. There is no officially accepted definition for functional foods, according to the European Commissions Concerned Action on Functional Food Science in Europe. Functional foods can be considered those that, beyond the adequate effect of basic nutrition derived from protein, lipid and glucid adequacy in quantity, quality and caloric proportion and trace elements such as minerals and vitamins, contain chemical compounds that have scientifically demonstrated special beneficial effects on the structures and functions of organs and systems that optimize them. Beneficial effects related to modern knowledge on physiology and cellular metabolism, which translates into risk reduction of chronic diseases such as those mentioned, increase life expectancy and quality of life, by delaying the ageing process, an action called antiageing.

Below we transcribe the internationally accepted conditions to consider food functional·

a. It must produce beneficial physiological effects on the state of physical or mental health, and/or reduce the risk of disease.

b. The aforementioned health properties must be demonstrated on a solid and true scientific basis.

c. The food component responsible for its physiological effects must be characterized by physical and chemical properties, as well as identified and quantified by available analytical methods.

d. The mentioned compound must have been evaluated in human groups in relation to absorption, distribution, metabolism, excretion and the mechanisms of action.

e. It must be effective in all members of a population or specific group of it, which must be clearly defined, by age, genetic make-up and so on.

Many studies have been carried out on fruit and vegetables enriched by impregnation techniques with minerals, calcium and zinc, probiotics (mainly lactobacilli and bifidobacteria) and phenolic bioactive compounds[354-356] adding to the high protein value of meat, and functional foods that increase their nutritional value, mainly through antioxidants, fibre and other probiotics.[357]

Functional foods are effective in the general population, unlike diet foods intended for certain groups of people with pathophysiological characteristics, such as coeliacs or diabetics.

It is worth highlighting in this regard the role of composition and quality as much or more than the quantity of food to which it refers.

Foods that have been clearly shown to have functional actions are few: prebiotics, which are foods rich in fibre; probiotics, which are fermented foods and unpasteurized, such as the aforementioned virgin apple cider vinegar and fermented beetroot; foods rich in omega-3 lipid acids such as avocados, walnuts and especially fish and krill; virgin olive oil and wine, especially red wine in moderate quantities, due to the content of antioxidants and anti-inflammatory polyphenols and for the content of oleic acid in olive oil.

This being a new issue during the last three decades, as far as the food-producing industry is concerned, sufficient legislation and regulations have not yet been drawn up. It is necessary for the rigorous control of advertisements and the health and safety of products. Japan is the country that has made the most progress, while in Europe different countries are developing common criteria in this regard.

In Argentina, the National Food Commission works to develop methods that regulate the production of prebiotics and probiotics.

It should be noted that a diet based on various natural foods in their natural state, or that have not been subjected mainly to industrial processing, provides functional foods.

Prebiotics are those that favour the development of intestinal bacterial flora due to fibre content. Fibre present in vegetables and fruit, in addition to promoting the development of intestinal bacterial flora, has other important health effects. It stimulates intestinal transit which prevents constipation, consequently decreasing the contact time of faeces with the terminal intestinal epithelium. Fibre is also fermented by intestinal bacteria with the production of butyric acid, which does not exist in food and is the main nutrient of the enterocyte, the cell of the intestinal epithelium. This allows the intestine to function in the best possible way, for its double actions as a barrier for toxins and bacteria with its richness of lymphatic cells that makes it an important immune defence organ, and for the absorption of nutrients. Other fibre functions have been referred to in Chapter 3.

In addition to fibre as a prebiotic, the first and irreplaceable functional food is breast milk for its content of beta lactose that allows the development of the bacillus Bifidus, as opposed to the alpha lactose of cow's milk that induces the development of coli.

Breast milk should be considered a functional food due to its many benefits. Even in a hypothetical case, where the composition of breast milk is faithfully reproduced in cow's milk with all its plastic, energetic, mineral, vitamin, enzymatic, hormonal and immunological components, both cellular and humoral, it cannot be a substitute for breastfeeding.

It is thus worth noting that everything referred to as important health benefits of functional foods through control and modulation of metabolism and all systems: immune, endocrine, nervous, circulatory, respiratory, digestive and reproductive, applies not only to some products made by the food industry but fundamentally to certain natural foods. Even these natural foods are superior to commercial products, so they should be, if possible, preferred for consumption. As an example, in addition to breast milk compared to its substitutes, fruit and vegetables can be compared to foods made with antioxidant and fibre supplements.

Fruit and vegetables are functional foods that provide complex glucides with a low glycemic index, many of them little or not absorbable due to their high fibre content. The maturing and preservation of intestinal functions are achieved by butyric acid, the nutrient par excellence of the enterocyte, generated in the bacterial fermentation of fibre, which we can classify as the second great functional food.

In fruit and vegetables, lycopene has also been attributed as a functional food in the prevention of numerous diseases.

Probiotics are saprophytic bacteria that contribute to the body to enrich and favour the development of the intestinal bacterial flora itself, the microbiota, which with its microbiome incorporates essential nutrients for the integrity and function of the intestinal epithelium and epigenetic components that stimulate or inhibit translations of our genome. They also prevent the development of pathogenic bacteria. Probiotics have long been empirically incorporated into almost all populations through home manufacture of naturally fermented foods such as wine, vinegar and pickled beetroot.

Fermented beetroot of Slavic and Baltic origin is a popular drink in Russia and Ukraine, known as beetroot Kvass, as it is also made with various fruit and vegetables. Beetroot Kvass is symbiotic due to its properties as a probiotic as a result of fermentation and as a prebiotic due to its fibre content. It can be made at home as described in the final chapter and should be ingested on an empty stomach in a small glass of alcohol. It is convenient to complement the consumption of fermented beetroot with *beetroot juice* due to its content of vitamins, mainly vitamin B including B_9 or folate, vitamin C, minerals especially iron, magnesium, manganese and potassium; nitrates that the body transforms into nitrites, and anti-inflammatory and antioxidant phytochemicals, mainly betanin, scarce in other vegetables and responsible for the colour of beetroot. Consumption can be 200ml per day divided into three servings in between meals. In the case of sports practice or intense and prolonged exercise, consume two hours before the practice, at the end of it and one hour after dinner.

Glutamine, also present in beetroot is one of the few amino acids that contain two nitrogen atoms, an element of fundamental importance for cell structure and metabolic functions. It is involved in the synthesis of glutathione, mitochondrial biogenesis and the integrity of lymphocytes, monocytes and neutrophils and the enterocytes of the intestinal mucosa and muscle tissue. Consequently, it reinforces the immune system, the absorption of nutrients and the acid/base balance through renal ammonio genesis to eliminate hydrogen ions and preserves brain function by controlling the level of ammonia in the blood. Glutamine constitutes 60% of the amino acids in muscle tissue where it maintains glycogen concentration, improves contraction performance, maintains the acid/base balance by neutralizing lactic acid production and preserves tissue mass, avoiding sarcopenia. It is present in many foods of animal and vegetable origin, but it is lost during cooking, so is best obtained by the consumption of nuts, parsley, spinach and especially beetroot juice.

Nitrites, due to vasodilator action, lower blood pressure and increase blood flow, improving the supply of oxygen to cells with an ergogenic effect, which translates into greater efficiency and strengthening of muscle contraction and better cardiorespiratory performance.[358, 359]

Glucides of beetroot have a medium glycemic index of 61 and a glycemic load of 5, very low, so they do not influence the level of glycemia.

Oxalate content is significant, so excessive consumption should be avoided, which increases the risk of urinary stones. For this reason, if the recommended beetroot juice is consumed, the consumption of leaves should be avoided; they are edible but with an even higher content of oxalates.

Free radicals, oxidants and antioxidants

Atoms are made up of a central nucleus of particles with positive electric charge, the protons and an equal number of particles without electric charge, the neutrons, which together with protons determine the atomic weight. Around the nucleus, particles with a negative electric charge, electrons, rotate in the same number as protons.

In an organic system, the electrons in their orbits around the nucleus are commonly arranged in pairs.

Loss of an electron, which means oxidation, leaves an unpaired electron generating what is called a *free radical* and it is an *oxidant*. Loss of electrons from oxygen produces reactive oxygen species and there are also reactive nitrogen species derived from *nitric oxide* with antimicrobial action, and they are induced by cytokines, microbial products, lipopolysaccharides and interferon. Free radicals are very unstable, they seek to reconstruct the electronic pair, but since the electrons are not free, they take them from other substances in fractions of a second. The loss of electrons is called oxidation and the gain of electrons is called reduction. Oxidation-reduction (redox) reactions normally occur in cellular metabolism and are controlled by *antioxidants*, which release electrons, inactivating the free radicals, thus protecting proteins, lipids and DNA from oxidative damage. Fig. 7-3 The exaggerated production of free radicals and oxidative stress can occur among other situations for example, in nutritional deficits, infections, exaggerated sports practice, alcoholism, diabetes, xenobiotic abuse, liver damage and old age. They also increase due to cigarette smoking and radiation, and it is the cause of serious damage to organic cells.

Moderate oxidation, however, is useful to the immune system to attack pathogens and stimulate apoptosis, while intense oxidation causes the necrosis of cells. Oxidative stress is involved in the pathogenesis of many diseases, including neurodegenerative diseases such as Parkinson's, Alzheimer's or Huntington's, cardiovascular diseases, metabolic diseases due to oxidation of LDL cholesterol, cancer and ageing.

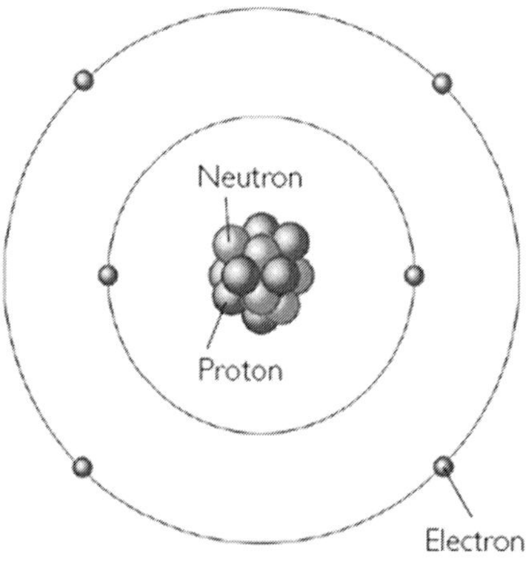

Protons: charges +. Electrons: charges

Fig. 7-2: Structure of an atom. Simplified bidimensional scheme

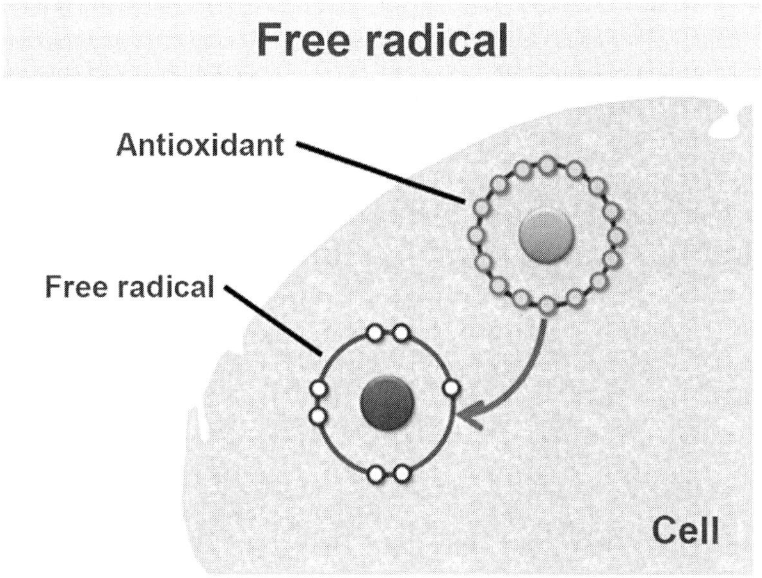

Fig. 7-3: Simplified bidimensional scheme

Antioxidants

Substances that neutralize the free radicals by giving up electrons protect cells from oxidative damage. These substances are antioxidants.

Endogenous antioxidants

Endogenous antioxidants typical of the body, are present in all cells and are supplemented with exogenous antioxidants present in some foods.

There are many situations in which the production of free radicals exceeds the neutralization capacity of endogenous antioxidants, hence the importance of supplementing meals with exogenous antioxidants.

The most studied are glutathione, coenzyme Q, catalase, peroxidase, superoxide dismutase and alpha-lipoic acid.

The most important is *glutathione*, 90 to 98% of which is in the form of reduced glutathione (GSH). Reduced glutathione acts as an antioxidant by giving electrons to free radicals and in the same way neutralising reactive oxygen and nitrogen species, thus preventing taking them from cellular proteins, with the consequent damage, which if it is important, can lead to cell death. By inactivating free radicals by giving them electrons, the reduced glutathione is left as oxidized glutathione disulfide (GSSG).

Oxidized glutathione is reactive but quickly combines with another and the reduced glutathione is regenerated. The GSH/GSSG index is an indicator of the degree of cellular toxicity. A low GSH/GSSG index occurs in oxidative stress.

It is the sulfhydryl (thiol) SH group of glutathione that acts as an electron donor. Glutathione is formed in the cytosol of cells, which is 80-85% of the total, 10-15% in the mitochondria and small percentages in the endoplasmic reticulum; the highest concentrations are in the liver. It is a tripeptide that results from 3 amino acids: glutamic acid, the sulfur amino acid cysteine and glycine. In its synthesis the enzyme glutamyl cysteine ligase intervenes, which is the limiting one, in addition to the fact that cysteine is scarce in food, then glutathione synthase acts. Glutathione is gamma L glutamyl L cysteine glycone.

In addition to precursors that come from proteins and are scarce when their digestion is difficult, such as antacids or antinutrients, vitamins B_6, B_9 and B_{12} are necessary. Lipoic acid and N acetylcysteine are also precursors, and their synthesis is increased by the action of curcumin. The antioxidant function is carried out by the action of the enzyme glutathione peroxidase and is reversed by reductase with NADH in the redox cycle. Glutathione increases the activity of all other antioxidants.

Due to oxidative stress, a decrease in GHS is observed in many diseases and this contributes to its worsening, as occurs in diabetes, liver disease, pulmonary fibrosis, poisoning, endotoxemia due to lipoperoxides and ageing. At the beginning of proliferative processes, GSH is located in the nucleus and regulates histone activity and influences DNA synthesis.

A high GSH/GSSH index regulates cell proliferation, apoptosis, immune functions, fibrogenesis, xenobiotic detoxification and delays ageing–the antiageing action.[360]

Exogenous antioxidants

Exogenous antioxidants, provided by various foods, are vitamins A, C, E and beta carotenes; the minerals copper, iron, manganese, zinc and selenium and phenolic compounds, flavonoids like quercetin and anthocyanins and non-flavonoids like tannins and lignans, or carotenoids without vitamin A activity like lycopene and a natural phenol, resveratrol. Glutathione is also present in fresh fruit and vegetables, spinach, avocado, nuts, tomatoes, grapefruit and other citrus fruit, berries, pomegranates, apples and watermelons, but with cooking it almost disappears.

Phenolic compounds constitute the natural defence of plants against predators and parasitism. They are present in cabbages, onion, garlic, carrot, mango, spinach, asparagus, blackberries, lemon, orange, virgin olive oil, green tea, yerba mate and wine. More than 10,000 phenolic derivatives are known, among them *flavonoids.*[361]

Flavonoids

They constitute a group of numerous substances synthesized by all plants, which protects them by antioxidant action from free radicals generated by ultraviolet radiation. The main flavonoids are quercetin, anthocyanin, naranginine, citrine, hesperidin, neohesperidin, flavones, isoflavones, catechin and epicatechin.

All are water-soluble polyphenols and have been extensively studied in their chemical structure and extraction media. Flavonoids derived from *flavus*, yellow, referring to the pigments of the vegetable kingdom, white as in onion, garlic, cauliflower or cabbage, green as in lettuce, spinach, arugula, broccoli or leek, yellow as in papaya, pear, citrus, plum or apricot, shades of orange to red such as orange, grapefruit, tangerine, radish, apple, beetroot, tomatoes–especially pearls or cherry. They are also present in grapes, red wine, beer, green tea, chamomile, yerba mate tea, cocoa, and chocolate with 70% cocoa and olive oil.[362] Flavonoids are believed to be primarily responsible for the therapeutic benefits of ginkgo Biloba, whose leaves turn intensely yellow in the autumn.

It should be highlighted first, as with other non-flavonoid phenols, its protective action against cellular oxidation by free radicals, generated by sunlight through ultraviolet rays, as well as by metabolism itself and especially in stressful situations such as intense exercise or illness, especially cancer, Flavonoids have anticancer and antiageing effects as well as antibacterial, antiviral and antifungal actions.

Among many flavonoids, *quercetin* will be mentioned first, which constitutes between 60 and 75% of all flavonoids present in food and is the one that has been studied the most in clinical evaluations. Studies carried out with quercetin do not show plasma levels after its ingestion, but high concentrations in tissues, mainly in the lung, liver, kidney and intestine and to a lesser extent in the brain. Free glycone is detected in plasma and vascular walls, a metabolite that is the end effector.[366, 367]

Regarding citrus fruit, Albert Szent-Gyorgyi saw that to reduce subcutaneous bleeding, lemon peel, due to the flavonoid citrin it contains, is more effective than pure vitamin C. In oranges, lemons and grapefruit they are mostly present in the peel. For this reason, the grating of whole oranges and lemons previously frozen in the freezer is particularly useful to add to soup, infusions and salads. For this, organic lemons or oranges are preferable as they have not been fumigated with insecticides or fungicides. Because flavonoids are sensitive to oxidation and heat, infusions such as tea, chamomile or ginkgo Biloba should be prepared at no more than 60º C. This is what the skin can endure for a short time without being damaged, the same is true for coffee. As for wine, it must be freshly opened, avoiding prolonged exposure to the air.

Two alcoholic drinks are especially rich in flavonoids, *limoncello* and *hesperidin.*

Limoncello, of Italian origin, is made with lemon peel, syrup and alcohol and is between 30 and 40% vol alcohol. Hesperidin is a liqueur created by Melville Sewell Bagley, an immigrant from Boston in the United States and the founder of the Bagley Company, and is made from bitter orange peel, a secret formula with 24 vol.% alcohol. Hesperidin was the first trademark registered in Argentina in 1864, awarded in the United States, Germany and France.

As a replacement for these alcoholic drinks, low-calorie drinks made with orange and lemon peel, as described in the final chapter, can be made at home.

Studies carried out with quercetin show its antioxidant, anti-inflammatory, and neutralizing action on advanced glycation products and excess estrogens.

Anthocyanins, especially in strongly coloured fruit such as berries, red apples, grapes and wine inhibit angiogenesis and tumour growth. Beneficial actions on the circulation have been proven. They act on the muscular layer of the vessels, increasing venous tone, improving return circulation and lymphatic drainage and reducing oedema. They improve endothelial function by increasing the synthesis of nitric oxide with a vasodilator effect, lower blood pressure in the presence of hypertension,[363,364] have antiatherosclerotic action[365]and inhibit platelet adhesion and aggregation by reducing the synthesis of thromboxane in platelets and leukotrienes in neutrophils with antithrombotic action. They also have anti-hemorrhagic action by reducing capillary permeability. The therapeutic benefits have been proven in purples of vascular origin, varicose veins, varicose ulcers and haemorrhoids.

Ongoing epidemiological studies seem to show a decreased risk of neurodegenerative and cardiovascular diseases, including myocardial infarction. They also have antiallergic and anticancer action.

Many flavonoid benefits postulated in various diseases can be attributed to their anti-inflammatory action, such as the reduction of pain observed in rheumatoid arthritis.

Non-flavonoids polyphenols

Non-flavonoid polyphenols are resveratrol, *cyanidin*, allicin, caffeine and gallic acid, rutin, myricetin, lignans and lycopene present in wine, cider, garlic and coffee.

Cyanidin is the most abundant. *Resveratrol* and the flavonoids catechin and epicatechin present in wine are the ones that have been studied the most. They are present more in red wine than in white because for the production of the latter the wine must be separated early from its skin, where these substances are mostly found. Catechin is found in a concentration of 191mg/litre in red wine and only 5mg/litre in white wine.

The protective effect of resveratrol on oxidative damage in the skin is induced not only by its action as an antioxidant but also by increasing endogenous antioxidants by activating glutathione synthesis.

Numerous antioxidants, including glutathione, resveratrol, vitamin C, hyaluronic acid and the fungus Ganoderma lucidum, have been studied for their protective action on the skin against injury from ultraviolet solar radiation. A decrease in the intracellular generation of reactive oxygen species produced by oxidative stress was observed, together with the activation of the epidermal stem cells, the protection of the extracellular matrix and immunomodulatory, antiallergic and antimicrobial action, preservation of histones and consequent stability of DNA with anti-ageing and anti-cancer properties.[368,369] They also protect coronary arteries improving cardiovascular function by antithrombotic, antihypertensive, anti-inflammatory, antioxidant action and a decrease in atherogenesis.[370,372] They can also increase bone mineralization reducing the risk of osteoporosis. Large prospective studies that demonstrate this benefit are still lacking.

Oxidative stress, due to an increased generation of free radicals, is created by air pollution, smoking, excessive alcohol, ultraviolet rays, diseases, especially cancer, intense exercise, advanced age or stress.[373] Antioxidants from food also act directly in the intestinal lumen on the oxidizing compounds present there.

Wine also has probiotic action due to naturally present lactic acid bacteria, resulting from malolactic fermentation that occurs once alcoholic fermentation is finished. These bacteria are resistant to saliva, acidity and bile salts and adhere to the mucosa of the digestive system, preventing the development of pathogenic bacteria, especially E coli.

Lignans

Lignans are also not flavonoid polyphenols but have a significant presence among phenolic compounds in olive oil, with their antioxidant action and anticancer action being evaluated.

Cancer cells produce a large number of reactive oxygen species that can act as inducers of cell growth factors. Knowledge of tumour cell biology shows genomic instability, resistance to chemotherapy and cancer activation induced by the persistent presence of free radicals. Lignans also block estrogenic effects, which gives them protective action against uterine, ovarian, prostate and breast cancer; they also activate enzymes for liver detoxification of xenobiotics.[374-378]

Lycopene

*Lycopene i*s a carotenoid without vitamin A activity. Like flavonoids, it protects plants from oxidation by sunlight in contact with air. It is a strong antioxidant, neutralizing free radicals and its action is twice as effective as vitamin E. It is present mainly in tomatoes and 10 times more in cherry tomatoes. It is in the red colouring of this and other fruit. The highest concentrations are in tomato sauce and fried tomatoes since lycopene is resistant to heat and is soluble in lipids. At high temperatures the membranes of the fruit break, releasing lycopene.

While the concentration of lycopene is 2mg% in fresh tomatoes, in fried tomatoes it is 25%. In addition, oil considerably increases its absorption, which in fresh tomatoes is only 3%.[379-381] But tomatoes should also be eaten fresh as flavonoids are sensitive to heat.

Lycopene is also present in watermelons, red grapefruit, apricots, pomegranates and peppers, but not in red peppers or cherries. It is also present in mushrooms and leafy vegetables, especially parsley.

|It is stored in many organs, mainly in the liver, lungs, prostate, colon, skin and cervix; organs in which anticancer action has been reported, but prospective studies are still lacking that demonstrate this.

Numerous studies have shown preventive action is twice as high as that of carotenes and anthocyanins on myocardial infarction.

Although studies are lacking to confirm this, a decrease in LDL and the prevention of arteriosclerosis, cataracts and macular degeneration, a frequent cause of blindness in the elderly, have also been reported. Evidence on stated benefits for asthma is also lacking.

Lycopene has other beneficial health effects, reducing the risk of numerous diseases. However, according to the Natural Medicines Comprehensive Database, which classifies efficacy based on scientific evidence, the action of lycopene is referred to as:

1. Ineffective in preventing bladder cancer and diabetes.
2. Insufficient evidence in relation to maculopathy, cataract, asthma, arteriosclerosis, gastric ulcer; cancer of the prostate, breast, uterus, cerebrospinal glioma, and colorectal; infection by the papillomavirus and hypercholesterolemia.
3. Epidemiological studies refer to the reduction of the risk of suffering from pancreatic cancer, cardiovascular diseases, atherosclerosis, hypertension and myocardial infarction, but other studies are discordant, or the benefits observed from the action of other components inherent in the consumption of fruits and vegetables cannot be defined.[382-384]
4. Predominantly with processed foods of high caloric density and poor nutritional value, the intake of lycopene and other natural antioxidants is insufficient. Most of the population does not meet a daily intake of

400 g. of fruit and vegetables, as recommended by the WHO. Given this, it is particularly useful to incorporate tomato fried in olive oil into the diet to increase the bioavailability and absorption of lycopene.[385]

Turmeric

Turmeric, also called Indian turmeric, Arab turmeric or eastern salt, has been used since ancient times in Indian and Chinese medicine. In India, for 6,000 years it was part of Ayurveda, the alternative herbal medicine integrated with the practice of yoga. In Japan, it is used with tea. It has curcumin diferuloylmethane, and golden spice turmeric, as the main of the three curcuminoids. Polyphenols are the active principles of the turmeric extract, which is obtained from the rhizomes of the roots of the Curcuma longa plant, of the ginger family, which is grown indoors as a houseplant.

On the packaging sometimes it is labelled as turmeric extract; in small quantities, it is found in condiments such as curries.

It is used as a condiment like ginger and as a nutritional supplement.

It contains Fe, Mn, vitamin B_6, and vitamin K and has strong antioxidant, anti-inflammatory and analgesic action, even referred to as superior in this regard to ibuprofen, hydrocortisone and chemotherapy drugs. It is not only highly effective but does not present undesirable side effects.

Curcuminoids have been approved by the American Food and Drug Administration as Generally Recognized as Safe and in clinical trials that have shown good tolerance and no toxicity, but they have poor bioavailability due to poor absorption and rapid metabolism.

With doses of 500 to 8,000mg. daily, no serum levels are detected, with 10 to 12g. low levels are detected, 50 ng./ml. low bioavailability for therapeutic effects, with excellent tolerance without toxic effects. But intakes greater than 8 g. are difficult. High doses can turn stools yellow.[386-389]

This has determined preparations with *nanocarriers*, and several components can increase bioavailability such as piperine, the active principle of black *pepper* that has been the most studied. It also increases solubility in alkalis, heat and oil and it is sensitive to light and should be stored in a refrigerator.

In humans, with the intake of 2g of curcumin alone, serum levels are not detected, or only scarcely, while together with 20mg of piperine, between 15 and 60 minutes after ingestion, increasing levels are observed by an increase of up to 2,000% of the bioavailability, which shows benefits in numerous diseases without adverse effects.[390]

Pepper

Black pepper, or piperine, acts as a bioavailability enhancer by action on absorption and metabolizing enzymes and exerts pharmacokinetic and pharmacodynamic interaction in medicinal co-administration, as with the use of nanocarriers of various materials being explored that allow easy absorption, dilution, transport and even cell penetration.

Nanocarriers generally are 1 to 100nm, and the limit is 1,000nm, with a large surface area in relation to volume.

Materials used are mainly lipids, crystals, gels, polymeric micelles, silica mesopores and proteins, such as ovalbumin, bovine serum albumin or casein.[391-398]

The first nanocarriers approved by the American Food and Drug Administration are liposomes made up of phospholipids, as cellular membranes. They are spherical vesicles, with nanoparticles of curcumin (Lipo-cur). Curcumin acts as anti-cytokines, such as TNFα and IL 1 beta, thereby inhibiting the formation of thromboxane and leukotrienes. As an antioxidant, it is much more effective than vitamins C and E. Among other inflammatory processes, it is postulated to be useful in arthritis, pancreatitis, Crohn's disease and intestinal inflammation. As anti-inflammatory it has analgesic action, like corticosteroids and NSAIDs such as phenylbutazone, but without the side effects of these drugs.[399]

With turmeric extract, its efficacy as an anti-inflammatory and analgesic has been observed in knee osteoarthritis and the consequent improvement in mobility and gait is equal to that of ibuprofen and diclofenac. A systematic evaluation of studies carried out and a meta-analysis of randomized clinical trials support the efficacy of turmeric for the treatment of arthritis, but for definitive conclusions, a greater number of studies and a larger sample size are necessary.[400-402]

As an antiplatelet agent, it has anti-atherosclerotic properties, it also increases prostacyclins and lowers cholesterol.

Like polyphenols of cranberry, strawberries and spinach, it is an important epigenetic factor reducing the risk for the development of cancer, cataracts, arthritis and Alzheimer's disease.[403]

In cancer, its actions are those of a pleiotropic, anti-inflammatory and antioxidant compound and among other actions, it induces apoptosis, reverses resistance to chemotherapy drugs and modulates multiple molecular signalling pathways.[404,405]

In ophthalmology, a benefit has been observed in anterior uveitis, age-related macular degeneration, diabetic retinopathy, glaucoma and dry eye syndrome.[406]

Among the numerous beneficial effects for health, in addition to those already mentioned, protective action against radiation damage, heavy metal poisoning and the destruction of cancer cells, reversing resistance to chemotherapeutic agents, has been enunciated, also its neuroprotective, anti-amyloid and antidepressant action.[407]

Nanoformulations with curcumin and various drugs enhance therapeutic effects and are still under investigation for large-scale production.[410-414]

An extensive review of the multiple beneficial actions for health from the numerous phytochemicals present in turmeric has recently been carried out in more than a hundred clinical tests on more than 1,000 patients. Turmeric extract contains several chemical constituents in addition to the polyphenols with the three curcuminoids, of which curcumin makes up about 90%. It also contains diterpenes, triphones, sterols and alkaloids. Their activities are not dependent on curcumin, a highly pleiotropic molecule. It has beneficial effects on irritable bowel syndrome, psoriasis, acne, vitiligo, gastric ulcer, lupus nephritis, chronic bacterial prostatitis, biliary dyskinesia, lipid metabolism and weight gain.[408-410]

In obesity, there is a state of oxidative stress and mild chronic inflammation that intervenes in the determining metabolic alterations of various diseases such as type 2 diabetes, hypertension, cardiovascular disease and various types of cancer. Turmeric in combination with piperine, due to its antioxidant and anti-inflammatory action, favours the reversal of metabolic syndrome by attenuating insulin resistance and thus hyperglycemia. Attenuation of the gene expression of hepatic lipogenesis and inflammation of the adipose tissue with decreased CRP and regulation of leptin and adiponectin secretion has been observed.[411-413]

It has anti-infective action by inhibiting the growth of pathogenic bacteria, viruses and fungi. Recently, effective action has also been observed on dengue virus and Covid 19.[414,415]

Turmeric also behaves as fibre and consequently with prebiotic action. It is not only digested by lactobacilli and bifid bacteria but also supports the growth of these bacteria and exerts a suppressive effect on the production of IL 8, a cytokine that is induced by lipopolysaccharides.[195]

Ginger

Linked to the turmeric family, *ginger* has more than 14 bioactive compounds, including gingerol, which has been the most studied. Observational studies in clinical and experimental animals show strong antioxidant, anti-inflammatory, anticancer, analgesic and antibacterial activities. It is a regulator of lipid metabolism and has protective effects on atherosclerosis and hepatotoxicity of ethanol. As an antioxidant, it inhibits superoxide production, suppresses lipid peroxidation and preserves reduced glutathione. It inhibits prostaglandins and leukotrienes and with fibrinolytic action reduces aortic atheroma. Studies on experimental animals, cell lines and others in vitro show that with ginger, pepper and turmeric there is an increase in length and perimeter of the *intestinal villi* in the small intestine, which increases the absorptive surface together with an increase in enzymatic activity of the intestinal membrane, with a consequent increase of micronutrient bioavailability.[420,421]

Saffron

Saffron is obtained from the stem stigma of the crocus sativus flower. Originating three or four thousand years ago from Egypt, Iran, Morocco, Greece and India, it is also produced in Spain, Great Britain and some European countries. From 25 tons of flowers, 1kg of saffron is yielded. Its use is almost exclusively in gastronomy due to its colour and aroma, and it is also used in the manufacture of some liqueurs.

As for its medicinal properties, it has been referred to as an antioxidant, a cytotoxic for cancer cells and is an anticonvulsant, an anti-depressant and a hypotensor.[422,423]

After analyzing the purity of the product used, scientific studies have been carried out on biological activities with possible therapeutic implications. In vitro studies have demonstrated antioxidant activity and in vivo, antineoplastic action has been demonstrated in rats with highly metastatic melanomas. The high cost of saffron compared to Curcuma and ginger, which share beneficial biological actions for health, limits its use as a nutritional supplement, being fundamentally of interest in gastronomy.

Chamomile tea

Chamomile is the opposite of caffeine, a relaxant recommended to be taken before going to sleep. It contains phytochemicals with antiestrogenic action. The crucifers broccoli, cauliflower and Brussel sprouts also have this antiestrogenic action. Estrogenic compounds are present in beer, herbicides, pesticides, petroleum-derived chemicals and household cleaners: they are xenoestrogens and determine the accumulation of abdominal fat and gynecomastia in men.

Elemental chemistry of Polyphenols

Among phytochemicals, to determine the special importance of the *polyphenols* contained in vegetables, fruit and derivatives, such as oils and infusions, for the preservation of health and prevention and co-contributing treatment of numerous diseases, it is necessary to know the elemental chemistry of these products. Polyphenols are derivatives of *benzene*, a 6-carbon hydrocarbon, (C_6H_6) in a hexagonal ring with alternating double bonds. Its derivative with the addition of an O, substituting an H for an OH, is *phenol* or phenic acid (C_6H_6O). Fig. 7-4. Substituting H for OH at two or more carbons or also joining two or three phenolic rings we have the various polyphenols, for example, *resveratrol* ($C_{14}H_{12}O_3$) with two rings linked by ligation with two C.

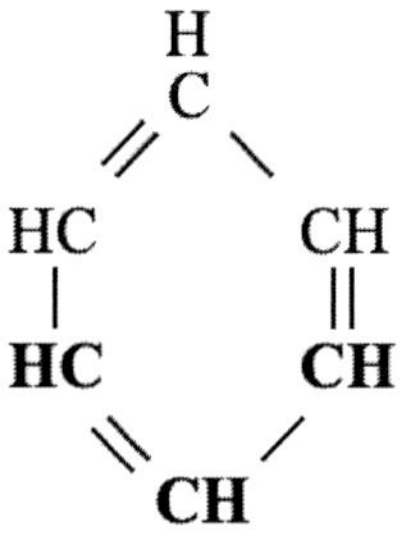

Bencene

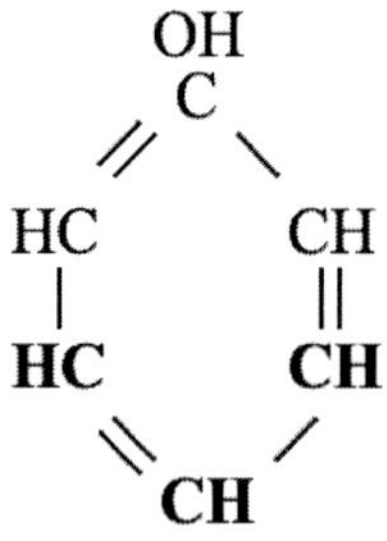

Phenol

Fig. 7-4

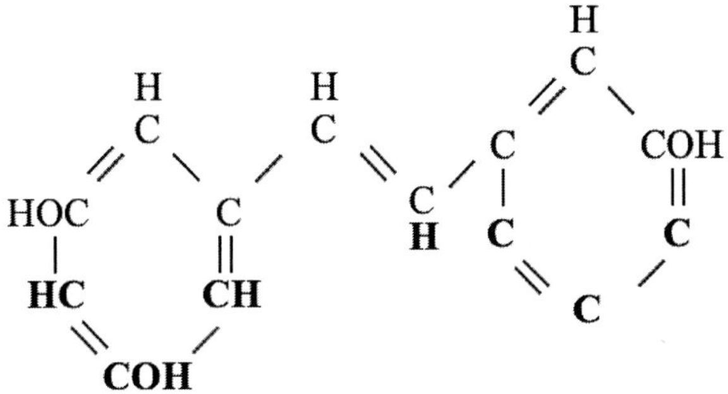

Resveratrol

Fig.7-5

Folate

Fruit and vegetables are also functional foods due to their content of *folate*, which is vitamin B_9. In the United States flour has been supplemented with folic acid since 1998, a synthetic product made by Lederle Laboratory in 1947, which is transformed into folate in the liver. For this reason, the particular folic acid supplement cannot be considered as a functional food but rather as a medicine to compensate for the low folate intake of diets with little vegetable intake and abundant processed foods.

The supplement of 1mg. or more of folic acid, is indicated for women from three months before and throughout pregnancy to prevent neural tube closure defects, such as myelomeningocele.

Mutations are currently known in the genotype of the enzyme *MTHFR* with reductions to 30-40% or 60-70% of the enzymatic activity in heterozygous or homozygous respectively, which interfere with the metabolism to convert folic acid into folate (vitamin B_9) and to convert homocysteine to methionine. Vitamins B_6 and B_{12} are also necessary for this. This can have important repercussions on development, chromosomal stability and variable interactions with carcinogenic mechanisms.

Elevated *homocysteine* levels are associated with an increased risk for cardiovascular disease if the level of 15uM/L is exceeded. This risk is mild with levels 15-30, intermediate 30-100, and severe with more than 100uM/L and is controlled or attenuated with strengthening or supplementation strategies.

It is different to increasing the supply of folates through the intake of appropriate foods, or the supply of L methyl folate already available in the United States than supplementing the diet with the supply of folic acid.

Folic acid is an artificial product that is transformed into folate in the liver; if liver capacity is saturated, unused folic acid can lead to numerous health problems such as leukaemias, arthritis, colorectal cancer and ectopic or multiple pregnancies.[424]

Regular consumption of various herbs with polyphenols with known beneficial effects on health reduces the risk of various diseases, but the concentration of active ingredients varies according to the age of the plants, the time of year and soil moisture among other factors and the preparation of infusions or other forms of consumption. Fresh vegetables and fruit with a low degree of maturity have higher polyphenols content. Work is being done with extracts of active ingredients feasible for dosage for therapeutic applications.

Sufficient and effective folate supply can be achieved by incorporating foods with high folate content (Table 7-1) into our usual meals, which must be consumed fresh and without cooking, otherwise, folate content is very significantly lost. Folate is stored in the liver, so daily intake is not necessary. A child requires 200ug daily which can come from one avocado and orange. An adult requires 400ug and 600ug in pregnancy. Other foods, without discarding them, can be complementary because with cooking the preferred content is only approximate; it may be less depending on the cooking mode and time. Liver contains 217ug.% of folate and can be supplied once or twice a week in part as a replacement for red meat along with broccoli, cooked for two minutes by blanching or steaming, with mushrooms.

One avocado	154
Turnip greens, 14g	106
Spinach, lettuce, 14g	58
One orange	40
Almonds, 150g	54

Table 7-1: Food with the highest folate content (ug).

When folate is precisely indicated, it should not be replaced by folic acid.

Conjugated linoleic acid

Based on studies originally on animals, *conjugated linoleic acid* has been attributed almost innumerable possible beneficial properties for health such as the prevention of cardiovascular disease, anticancer action, especially for prostate, colon, skin and breast, antidiabetic action improving insulin sensitivity, reducing body fat, reducing adiposity in obese patients and reducing weight gain, especially due to the action of the 10-trans 12-cis isomer, which is not the most abundant.

It was also noted that increased protein synthesis in muscle tissue and bone mineralization prevent sarcopenia and osteoporosis, and the transport of calcium to the joint cartilage would have anti-inflammatory action. If these effects also occurred in humans, this would be useful in sport.

Possible modulatory effects of the immune system and anti-inflammatory action with potential usefulness for inflammatory bowel disease, Crohn's disease and food allergies were mentioned with stimulation of IgA, IgG and IgM and a decrease of IgE.[425]

Observations made with randomized studies with double-blind controls give different actions according to isomers used, with opposing effects on LDL, HDL and total/HDL (Castelli index) cholesterol depending on whether cis-9 trans-11 or trans-10 cis-12 isomer is used.[426-428]

Conjugated linoleic acid produced naturally by ruminates, present in milk and meat from grass-fed animals, is saturated lipid acid with beneficial effects on health, but due to the isotopes present it is different from that achieved by hydrogenation, with effects that are controversial and may even be harmful.

No undesirable effects have been reported with intakes of up to 7.2g per day. For the Food and Drug Administration, it is generally recognized as safe in 60 to 90% of a mixture of cis-9, and trans-11, in a ratio of 50:50.

A common Western diet can provide anywhere from 150 to 200mg. to 1.5g. per day. It is said that to obtain beneficial effects, 2 to 3 g. per day or more should be ingested. Consumption of 6g. per day for 1 year or 3.4g.

for 2 years is effective for reducing body mass, with results already observed at 6 months with 3.2 to 3.4g. per day.[429-431]

CHAPTER 8

COMPLEMENTARY HEALTH HABITS

Intermittent fasting

With studies on experimental animals and humans, beneficial health effects have been documented with *intermittent fasting,* to be practised three or four times a year or even more frequently according to medical indications. We can practice the same after eating breakfast without net glucides or meat, chicken or fish.

For breakfast: a handful of green leaves with chopped fruit with olive oil and apple cider vinegar (manufactured as described later), and then two eggs with butter. After this, the fast is fulfilled for 24 or 48 hours with only the ingestion of water in infusions preferably of Yerba Mate tea, green tea or vegetable broth, amounting to approximately seven servings of 250ml.

This causes a slight decrease in weight, increases sensitivity to insulin and leptin, normalizes levels of ghrelin (the hunger hormone) which slows ageing and burns fat, reduces oxidative stress and free radicals and lowers LDL cholesterol and triglycerides. With intermittent fasting, a decrease in inflammatory processes, a reduction in blood pressure, an improvement in cardiac and cerebral functionalism, an increased resistance to cancer and neurodegenerative diseases, such as Parkinson's, Alzheimer's and Huntington's, and the prevention of brain volume and weight loss is observed, that is usually seen with senescence.

Benefits observed at the cellular and molecular level are similar to those resulting from regular physical exercise and its mechanism seems to be related to a decrease in oxidative damage and an increase in cellular resistance to stress, mediated among other factors by the protective action of champerone proteins, such as those released in heat shock, described later.[432-434]

Avoid sedentary lifestyle

Active exercise stimulates the production of new brain cells, just like coffee and turmeric raise the level of neurotrophic factors derived from the brain. Biogenesis and mitochondrial activity are also activated by this factor. The most ancestral and aerobic thing is to walk in an environment of pure air, walk or run through a park, through a field or street enjoying the air, the sun and nature. When possible, climb stairs instead of using the lift or escalators.

Avoiding a sedentary lifestyle can also mean Swedish gymnastics, (without apparatus), or a current version of it, such as the fashionable9-minute system that will be discussed later.

Exercise of a certain muscle group increases blood flow with a local increase in lipolysis in the adjacent cell tissue. This seems to be mediated by systemic epinephrine and norepinephrine increase with higher local concentrations due to an increase in blood flow in the area of muscular exercise.[435]

For those who have the inclination and opportunity a moderate practice of sports, such as swimming, rowing, tennis or golf that do not pose major health risks due to accidents is also recommended for their physical and social implications.

Sports such as football, rugby, horse riding or as is currently in vogue, running long distances, have other motivating factors beyond those strictly related to health.

These sports practices, due to accidents or overexertion involve the risks of tendonitis, joint pain, sprains, dislocations, muscle tears, bone fractures or visceral trauma.

Gymnastics in 9 minutes

This is based on the high-intensity circuit training, developed by Chris Jordan, Director of Exercise at the Physiology Human Performance Institute and consists of a series of 13 exercises (Fig. 8-1) each of which is practised for 30 seconds, with 10 seconds of rest between each.

The timing of the exercises and rest between each is controlled by counting 1001, 1002, and 1003 until 1010 and continuing with 11, 12 and 13 up to 30 for exercises and until reaching 1010 for the breaks.

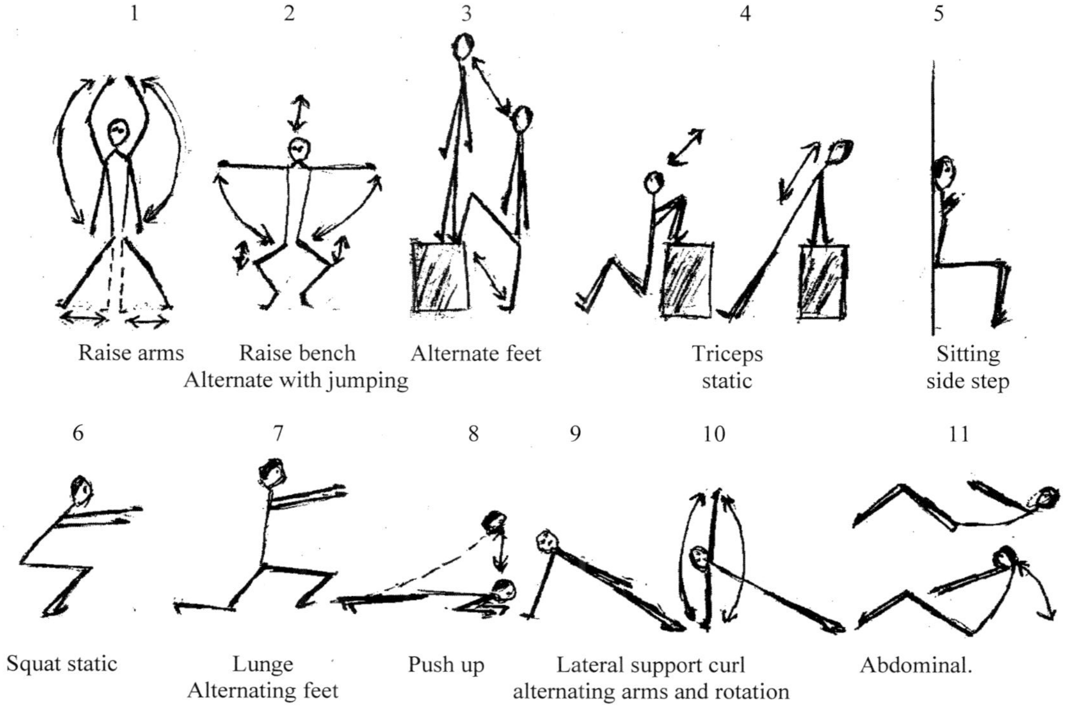
1
Raise arms
2
Raise bench
Alternate with jumping
3
Alternate feet
4
Triceps
static
5
Sitting
side step
6
Squat static
7
Lunge
Alternating feet
8
Push up
9
10
Lateral support curl
alternating arms and rotation
11
Abdominal.

12 13

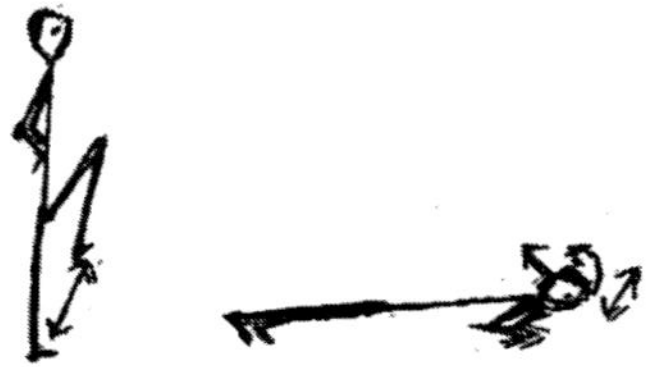

Alternating Static leaning on elbows and feet

Fig. 8-1: Gymnastics in 9 minutes
Based on the High-Intensity-Circuit-Training, H.I.C.T, by Chris Jordan

They are practised daily or at least five days a week indoors or outdoors.

They exercise a large part of the muscle groups and mobilize numerous joints, many of which are often not activated in daily life. They activate the respiratory and cardio-circulatory systems, stimulate metabolism and maintain muscle tone and mass.

Depending on the initial physical state and training achieved, after weeks or months, if a greater intensity is desired, exercises can be practised for 40 seconds, which extends the duration of the entire series to 11 or 12 minutes.

Exercise Two can become the last one and is practised for 45 seconds, as an intense and short-duration exercise. It can cause anaerobiosis with elevated lactic idemia, and the aforementioned lactic acidosis, an important means of hormonal stimuli with cardiac tonic and antiageing effects.

After exercise, shower with hot water for two or three minutes, with soap only for the perineal area. Then continue to shower for 1 minute with cold water. A 4ºC. drop in skin temperature releases heat shock proteins. Wash the hair two or three times a week

In sports training, muscle inflammation resulting from exercise is a favourable factor in promoting muscle development, to which the action of arachidonic acid from the aforementioned protein sources can be added, recommended within 30 minutes after exercise, the moment of greatest avidity for tissue replenishment..

Heat shock proteins

Heat shock proteins belong to the group of stress proteins. Several of the aforementioned champerones are known, among the main ones, are four variables of heat shock proteins, the protein associated with the receptor for tumour necrosis factor-alpha, proteins regulated by glucose and others.

In exercise 13, do 10 seconds of cervical flexion and extension, 10 seconds with cervical twists to the right and left and 10 seconds with cervical flexions on the left and right shoulder. In addition, in exercise 14, with the arms behind the neck, alternately touch the elbows with the contralateral knees while extending the lateral leg.

Champerones produced by all cells are the most conserved proteins in both prokaryotic and eukaryotic cells with different functions depending on their location, within the cell or on the cell membrane. They are expressed against harmful physiological or environmental agents such as cytotoxins, acidosis, infections or inflammatory processes, increasing the capacity for survival and adaptation to adverse conditions. These stress proteins, or heat shock, bind to nascent peptides directing folding and then conservation of the three-dimensional structure of amino acids for the function of proteins, and interact in the modulation of *apoptosis* together with mitochondrial action. In cell membrane, they exert immunological functions avoiding hyperactivity of inflammation.

Apoptosis plays a fundamental role in maintaining a state of cellular health both in development and in immune defences and is regulated by pro and anti-apoptosis factors. Dysregulation of apoptosis isan important factor in the origin and evolution of various diseases. Due to the leading role in apoptosis of

heat shock proteins, their stimulation has therapeutic implications.[436]

Heat shock proteins are being evaluated in preventive or curative actions on atheroma plaques in vascular walls and experimental studies seem to show implications in the protection of intestinal epithelium against aggression by lectins.[437,438]

The pleiotropic functions of heat shock proteins are presented with therapeutic perspectives in cancer and kidney diseases.[439-441] Possible protective action against neurodegenerative diseases, such as Parkinson's and Huntington's, named conformational diseases or proteinopathies, due to alterations in the three-dimensional structure of amino acid chains, has been reported.

Breathing

Breathing should always be nasal; the nose warms and moistens the air and respiratory cilia purify the air by trapping impurities. It favours lung elasticity due to the smaller calibre of the nasal airway when compared to oral respiration. Nasal mucosa synthesizes nitric oxide that passes into the blood and exerts vasodilator and bronchodilator effects. Oral breathing aggravates asthma, especially that triggered by exercise.[442]

Breathing should be smooth inspiration and expiration almost without noticing thoracic or abdominal excursion. Deep breathing, as people generally do when exercising, talking, sighing or yawning, eliminates excess CO_2 which reduces the release of O_2 from oxyhaemoglobin to the tissues (the Bhor effect) with vasoconstriction and an elevation of blood pressure.

An increase in CO_2 tolerance increases exercise endurance and improves cellular oxygenation.

Tolerance to CO_2 can be measured in seconds. Sitting without crossing your legs, breathe gently and after an exhalation, hold your nose and take the time until you feel the need to breathe, this can manifest itself with contractions of the chest or abdomen muscles. If the elapsed time is 40 to 60 seconds, there is excellent resistance to exercise and breathing is optimal. From 20 to 40 seconds there is a mild respiratory disorder and if it is from 10 to 20 seconds there is a serious respiratory disorder and little tolerance to exercise.

The state of respiratory function can be improved by doing the aforementioned exercise and repeating it every 20 or 30 seconds.

CHAPTER 9

RECIPES

Limoncello

This can be made with the peel of 10 lemons in 1 litre of alcohol and 3 litres of water with 800g. of honey. Leave for 10 days stirring every day, and filter.

Naliric

This alcoholic drink can be prepared with the peel of 10 lemons and 10bitter oranges in 1 litre of spirits, with 5g. of turmeric, 2 sprigs of rosemary, 4 sage leaves, 12g of black pepper and 8 cloves. Leave for 10 days stirring every day, filter and add 3 litres of water with 800g of honey. In this way, we have a drink that combines the properties of oranges, lemons, honey, and the aforementioned herbs and reduces the alcohol content to about 25% vol. (15g%)

Virgin apple cider vinegar

Procedure

Boil 2 litres of water to remove the chlorine and add 2 teaspoons (5g each) of salt to prevent the development of pathogenic bacteria. Take two large red apples, with the peel cut into pieces without the core or seeds. When the water is cold or warm, place it with the apple pieces in the blender. Once blended, transfer to a wide-mouthed bottle and cover with a paper napkin so that it stays in contact with the air and keep it at room temperature.

Every day for a month, you should stir with a spoon and replace the cover with a paper napkin. At the end of the month, transfer to two bottles, one with a corrugated cork for consumption and the other for storage in the cupboard, always at room temperature. The bottle should be shaken every time before serving the vinegar. When starting the consumption of the one in storage, it should be prepared again at 1 or 2 litres.

You will be able to appreciate that the vinegar that has been in storage has stronger organoleptic characteristics, smell and taste and it also has stronger biological properties.

Almond milk

With 15 almonds per 150ml of water, add 5ml of olive oil with a teaspoon plus another teaspoon of glucose, or for children over 2 years, a teaspoon of honey.

Fermented beetroot

The preparation of 1 litre of fermented beetroot is carried out with a large beetroot from which the roots and residual shoots are removed, washed under running water and scrubbed with a metal sponge to remove any residual soil. Then it is divided into small pieces 2 or 3cm long and 1 cm thick that are placed in a wide-mouthed jar. Boil a litre of water to remove the chlorine. Once it is cold or warm add5g of salt, equivalent to a level teaspoon, to avoid the development of pathogenic bacteria. This water is added to the wide-mouthed jar where the beetroot chunks have been placed. Stir with a long-handled wide spoon then cover the mouth with a paper napkin. Shake every day for seven days. On the first day, white supernatant can form which can be removed with a strainer and discarded, it does not matter if there is some left as it will disappear when mixing.

After seven days, the liquid is transferred to a bottle with a lid, and this is put in the refrigerator. Drink 15 or 20ml daily on an empty stomach. The beetroot chunks left in the wide-mouth jar are thrown away or can be used for one more preparation.

Gelatin from bone broth

Steam 2 or 3kg of pork legs for 3 hours or cook in a pressure cooker with the valves at 60°. Then separate the legs for usual consumption and once the broth has cooled, place it in the refrigerator. Portions of that gelatin can be added to soups. It has the components of connective tissue: hyaluronic acid and chondroitin sulphate.

Broccoli, for sulforaphane production

Sulforaphane production is increased by putting all the chopped broccoli flowers in a container with 100g. of mustard dissolved in 250ml of water, mixing and letting it rest at room temperature for between 30 and 60 minutes, so that the myrosinase enzyme from the mustard acts on the glucoraphanin in the broccoli, producing sulforaphane. Then it must be steamed for 2 or 3 minutes, or by blanching adding 500ml of boiling water and leaving for 30 minutes, then cool it in the freezer for 90 minutes, without freezing it and keep it in the refrigerator. The reason for this procedure is that the enzyme myrosinase is sensitive to heat, unlike sulforaphane, which is resistant to heat. Conserve in a refrigerator and consume two or three times a week, cold or slightly warmed. From one head of broccoli, you can get five or six servings.

Vegetable omelette

Ingredients

2 bundles of spinach, leek or chard
2 cloves of garlic
4 eggs
Black pepper to taste
Vegetable spray or olive oil

Method:

Chop the vegetables and garlic very small.
Place them in a bowl, add the eggs and season.
Mix everything and separate into two equal portions.
Put each portion in a frying pan sprinkled with the vegetable or olive oil and cook on both sides.
The vegetable omelette can be used as a pizza base.

Green pizza

With one vegetable omelette instead of flour

Preparation of the sauce:

Ingredients

1 tomato
1 red bell pepper
Half an onion

Method:

Chop the tomato, bell pepper and onion.
Season to taste.
Fry with olive oil.

Place the sauce on the omelette and add chopped fresh tomato, cream cheese and to taste: ham, sardines or anchovies, mushrooms or artichoke hearts.

Cook in the microwave until the cheese is melted.

Aubergine Lasagna

Ingredients

1 kg. of aubergines
2 eggs
10 g minced garlic
10 g chopped parsley
A little salt and pepper
300 g grated cheese
200 g of flour
200 g of breadcrumbs
Ketchup
500 g. tomato puree
3 onions
A little bit of salt
A little oregano

Method

Peel the aubergines and cut lengthwise into thin slices.
Sprinkle the slices with coarse salt and leave for one hour.
Wash and dry with kitchen paper.

Roll the slices in the flour and then the beaten eggs, season with a dessert spoon (10g) of minced garlic and parsley and a little salt and pepper and then roll in the breadcrumbs.
Leave in the refrigerator for 30 minutes.
Cook in an oiled oven dish.
Peel the onions and chop them small; place them in a pan with oil to sautethem, then add tomato sauce, season with oregano, salt, garlic and parsley until the onion is cooked.

Reserve.

Place a little of the tomato sauce in an oiled baking dish, and then place some slices of the aubergines already cooked in the oven. Alternate aubergines and tomato sauce and finally put grated cheese on to brown in the oven.

Tripe stew

Makes 10 servings

Ingredients

1 red chorizo
1kg of tripe
2 large onions
2 carrots
1 red bell pepper and 1 green
200g bacon
500g tomato slices
3 large sweet potatoes
2 litres of vegetable broth

Method

Put the tripe in a pot covered with water and boil for two hours, remove, rinse and cut into cubes.
Sauté the onion and the chopped bell peppers, and season to taste.
Add chopped carrot.
Cook the bacon and diced chorizo together with the tripe for a few minutes.
Add the tomato, seasonings and broth, lower the heat, cover and cook for sixty minutes and add the sweet potato and pumpkin until they are cooked.

To serve.

The tripe can be replaced by roast beef.

Stuffed courgettes

Ingredients

6 round courgettes
2 onions
1 clove garlic
Half a red bell pepper
9 eggs
Grated cheese, salt, pepper

Method

Steam the courgettes for 20 minutes, then cut them in half and place them upside down to drain.
Chop onion, garlic and bell pepper very small and sauté in a pan.
Remove the pulps from the courgettes and place them together with the onions, season, add the eggs and mix until smooth.
Fill the courgettes and place grated cheese on for browning.
Put the courgettes in the preheated oven for 10 minutes until they are au gratin.

Cauliflower or broccoli with white sauce

Ingredients

2 cauliflowers
White sauce:
100g butter
100g flour
1 litre of milk
Nutmeg
Salt and pepper to taste
Grated cheese

Method

Steam the cauliflower for 20 minutes. Reserve.
In a saucepan melt the butter over medium heat and add the flour.

Let the mixture cook for a minute, stirring all the time with a wooden spoon, then remove the saucepan from the heat and add a little milk.
Continue mixing until everything is integrated, then add the remaining milk little by little, always mixing.
To finish, put it back on the heat and add nutmeg, salt and pepper, continue mixing until you get a thick sauce. Reserve.
Place the cauliflower pieces in a baking dish, add the white sauce until it covers everything and add the grated cheese.
Cook in the oven for 15 minutes until au gratin.

Catalan salad

Ingredients

1 aubergine, 1 onion and 1 red bell pepper

Method

Roast them whole in the oven until they become soft, peel them and cut them into thin strips.
Add olive oil and virgin apple vinegar and season with pepper and salt.

Roast

Be it beef, lamb or suckling pig, instead of grilling horizontally over the embers, it can be done almost vertically on the grill and although it takes much longer (up to three or four hours), this is healthier because it is at a lower temperature that never reaches 38ºC and the juices do not fall on the embers giving off carcinogenic fumes. If the meat is first drizzled with apple cider vinegar, this moderates glycation even more, although it also attenuates the rich taste that originates with glycation.

Turmeric applications

Add turmeric to your salad to give it a bolder yellow colour, or season it with turmeric, cumin and coriander.

For a creamy and rich sauce mix a little turmeric and dried onion with a little mayonnaise, salt and pepper.

To dress salads: four tablespoons of olive oil, a tablespoon of lemon juice, two of orange juice and a pinch of black pepper. Prepare at the time of serving so as not to lose the vitamin C in the juice. It is a sauce that is truly natural medicine; it brings together a series of foods, all of them especially anti-cancer: turmeric, vitamin C, vitamin E and omega-3 from olive oil, also favourable for preventing cardiovascular diseases.

Beetroot juice

One large beetroot, without leaves or roots, well washed, is cut into small cubes of 2 or 3 cm. and placed in a jar with a lid with 600ml of water and stirred with a spoon three times on the first day and stored in the refrigerator. From the next day, 100ml is taken on an empty stomach three times a day, having mixed with a spoon. If you do sport, one intake should be before and another after it, and the last one before going to bed.

Juices with two or three vegetables and fruit:

You can use spinach, carrot, lettuce, arugula, strawberries, avocado, orange, lemon, banana, or others according to taste and can you also add a little ginger.

A smoothie of this type can be made, for example for three people, with half a carrot, half a cucumber, 3 broccoli flowers, a lettuce leaf and an orange with two glasses of water.

Parsley tea

The water should be boiled and then add the parsley (a teaspoon, 5g or more) and leave for 20 minutes. Add 2g of ginger and 2g of cinnamon.

GLOSSARY

Covalent bonds

Are unions of elements, not by difference in electric charge, but by shared electrons; these types of unions are common in organic chemistry and break by oxidation releasing large amounts of energy.

Glycosides

When glucids are linked to substances of another chemical nature, in these compounds the glucid receives the name of glycone and the other substance that of aglycone.

Flavonic glycosides have as aglycon a flavonoid, rutin, quercetin and hesperidin, with antioxidant action and some with the property of reducing capillary fragility.

Cardiotonic glycosides, as digitalis from the purple digitalis plant (foxglove).

Cyanogenetic glycosides in fruit seeds, bitter almonds, pulses and cassava, by the action of the cyanide glucosidase enzyme, can inhibit cellular respiration and lead to death. Subsequent soaking and cooking will remove hydrocyanic acid.

Terpene glycosides and steroids are saponins capable of producing hemolysis and intestinal damage, apparently not active orally and mostly inactivated by heat.

Glycoproteins are the lectins or hemagglutinins present in pulses, mostly inactivated by heat.

Heteropolysaccharids

Have different monosaccharides, which are repeated in alternating order, some with groups of different chemical structures, amines, sulfates, or chains of amino acids (polypeptides). These are essential structural components of tissues related to cell walls and extracellular matrices. They also modulate communication between the cell and secretion cells that plug wounds in plants and in the saliva of sucking insects, preventing blood clotting.

Agar-agar Pectins

Rubber bands

Hemicellulose

In higher animals, mucopolysaccharides or glucose-amino-glucans

Hyaluronic acid, a component of connective tissue

Chondroitin, a component of cartilage

Heparin, in the liver and lungs.

Homopolysaccharide

Are made up of the union of the same monosaccharide

BIBLIOGRAPHY

1. Interview by Dennis Hughes of Share Guide with Jack LaLanne (1914-2011).
2. Cordain L. "Jack LaLanne´s story." *The Paleo Answer* Ed. John Wiley & Sons Inc. 2012. Hoboken: New Jersey.
3. Katz D.L, Meller S. "Can We Say What Diet Is Best for Health?" *Annual Review of Public Health*. 2014; 35: 83-103.
4. Sandoval-Insausti H, Blanco-Rojo R, Graciani A, et al. "Ultra-processed Food Consumption and Incident Frailty: A Prospective Cohort Study of Older Adults." *Journal of Geront A BiolMed Sci*. 2020; 75:1126-33.
5. Wendel Berry. In: *Vida Natural y Orgánica*. 20 February 2015.
6. Pieczenik S.R, Neustadt J. "Mitochondrial dysfunction and molecular pathways of disease". *Exp Mol Pathol*. 2007; 83: 84-92.
7. Wallace D.C. "A mitochondrial paradigm of metabolic and degenerative diseases, ageing, and cancer: a dawn for evolutionary medicine." *Ann Rev Genet*.2005; 39: 359-407.
8. Uberos J. "Microbiota perinatal: Revisión de su importancia en la salud del recién nacido Perinatal microbiota: review of its importance in newborn health." *Arch Argent Pediatr*. 2020;118: e265-e270.
9. Loyacono N, Sanz M.L, Gerbi M.D y col. "Problemas gastrointestinales, nutricionales, endocrinológicos y de microbiota en el trastorno del espectro autista Gastrointestinal, nutritional, endocrine, and microbiotaconditions in autism spectrum disorder." *Arch Argent Pediatr*. 2020; 118: e271-e277.
10. Dupré J. "Más allá del Darwinismo." *Ciencia Hoy*. 2009; 19: 8-8.
11. Calvo E. Amamantamiento "¿Un lenguaje cifrado entre la madre y el niño?" *Boletín CESNI*: 1993; 6: 3-8.
12. Voyer L.E. "Introducción a la Pediatría." In: *Pediatría*. (Eds) Voyer, Ruvinsky, Cambiano. 3rd Ed. 2011, Ediciones Journal: Buenos Aires.
13. Lactancia Materna y Alimentación con Leche Humana. Documento Oficial de la Academia Americana de Pediatría de los Estados Unidos de América. Sección Lactancia. Pediatrics online. February 27, 2112; DOI: 10. 1542/peds. 2011-3552.

14. Brahm P, Valdés V. "Beneficios de la lactancia materna y riesgos de no amamantar." *Rev Chil Pediatr*. 2017; 88.
15. Stuebe A. "The risks of not breastfeeding for mothers and infants." *RevObstetGynecol*. 2009; 2: 222-31.
16. Código Internacional de Comercialización de Sucedáneos de la Leche Materna, (IBFAN- CP 157, 1211 Ginebra, Suiza). *Actualización* 2017.
17. Muzzio de Califano C, Ferrario C. "Lactancia materna." In Voyer LE, Ruvinsky R, Cambiano C. Pediatría. 3rd. Ed. *Ediciones Journal*. Buenos Aires. 2011.
18. Carlson S.E. "Docosahexaenoic acid and arachidonic acid in infant development". Seminars in Neonatology. 2002; 6: 437-49.
19. Vaarala O, Paronen J, Otonkoski T.A, et al. "Cow milk meals induces antibodies to insulin in children-a link between cow milk and insulin-dependent diabetes mellitus?" *Scand J Immunol*. 1998; 47: 131-5.
20. Vaarala O, Knip M, Paronen J, et al. "Cow's milk formula meals induces primary immunization to insulin in infants at genetic risk for type 1 diabetes". *Diabetes*. 1999; 48: 1389-94.
21. Writing Group for the TRIGR Study Group, Knip M, Åkerblom HK, et al. "Effect of Hydrolyzed Infant Formula vs Conventional Formula on Risk of Type 1 Diabetes: The TRIGR Randomized Clinical Trial." *JAMA*. 2018; 319: 38-48.
22. Hoyt G, Hickey M.S, Cordain L. "Dissociation of the glycaemic and insulinemic responses to whole and skimmed milk." *Br J Nutr*. 2005; 93: 176-7.
23. Rizza R.A, Mandanno L.J, Gemnest J, et al. "Production of insulin resistance by hyperinsulinaemia in man." *Diabetología*. 1985; 26: 70-5.
24. Maldonado Lozano D.J, MataixVerdú D.J. "Patología digestiva: Teoría y práctica clínica." Cap. 7. Malabsorción de hidratos de carbono. Pg. 135. En: *Asignatura Patología Digestiva*. FUNIBER. Maestría de Nutrición y Dietética. Univ. Europea Miguel de Cervantes. 2013.
25. Avila Castañón L, Hidalgo Castro E.M, del Río Navarro BE, et al. "Alergia a la proteína de la leche de vaca [Cow's milk's protein allergy]." *Rev AlergMex*. 2005; 52: 206-212.
26. Demis M, Loras-Duclaux I, Lachaux A. "Cow's milk protein allergy through human milk." *Arch Pediatr*.2012; 19: 305-12.

27. Aghasi M, Golzarand M, Shab-Bidar S, et al. "Dairy intake and acne development: A meta-analysis of observational studies." *Clin Nutr*. 2019; 38:1067-75.
28. Penso L, Touvier M, Deschasaux M, et al. "Association Between Adult Acne and Dietary Behaviours: Findings From the Nutri Net-Santé Prospective Cohort Study." *JAMA Dermatol*. 2020; e201602
29. Adebamowo C. A, Spiegelman D, Berkey C.S, et al. "Milk consumption and acne in teenaged boys." *J Am Acad Dermatol*. 2008; 58: 787-93.
30. Goldberg J.P, Folta S.C, Must A. "Milk: can a ''good'' food be so bad?" *Pediatrics*. 2002; 110: 826-32.
31. Oski F. "Does drinking milk help prevent osteoporosis?" In: *Don't drink your milk. Capítulo 6*. Pickle Pub. Minnesota. 2004.
32. Gil M.E. "Relación entre la problemática ambiental y la salud del niño." In: Voyer, Ruvisnki, Cambiano. *Pediatría* 3ª Ed. 2° tomo. 2011: 1373. Ed. Journal. BuenosAires.
33. Voyer L.E. "Presentación de la Segunda Edición de Criterios de Diagnóstico y Tratamiento." *Rev Pediatr Elizalde*. 2012; 3: 3-5.
34. Singla R, Garg A, Surana V et al. "Vitamin B12 Deficiency is Endemic in Indian Population: A Perspective from North India." *Indian J Endocr Metab*. 2019; 23: 211-14.
35. Basak T, Garg G, Bhardwaj N, et al. "Low holo-transcobalamin levels are prevalent in vegetarians and is associated with coronary artery disease in Indian population." *Biomarkers*. 2016; 21: 436-40.
36. Werder S.F. "Cobalamin deficiency: hyperhomocisteinemia and dementia." *Neuropsychiatr Dis Treat*. 2010; 6: 159-95.
37. Aguirre J.A, Donato M.L, Buscio M. y col. "Compromiso neurológico grave por déficit de vitamina B12 en lactantes hijos de madres veganas y vegetarianas." *Arch Argent Pediatr*. 2019; 117: e420-e424.
38. Famularo G, De Simone C, Pandey V, et al. "Probiotic lactobacilli: an innovative tool to correct the malabsorption syndrome of vegetarians?" *Med Hypotheses*.2005; 65: 1132-5.
39. Puppala K.R, Kumar V.R, Khire J., et al. "Dephytinizing and Probiotic Potentials of Saccharomyces Cerevisiae (NCIM 3662) Strain for Amelioration of Nutritional Quality of Functional Foods." *Probiotics Antimicrob Proteins*.2019; 11: 604-17.
40. VashishthA, RamS, Beniwa V, et al. "Cereal Phytases and Their Importance in Improvement of Micronutrient Bioavailability." Biotech. 2017; 7: 42.

41. Frolich W. "Chelating properties of dietary phytate. The role for bioavailability." *Adv Exp Med Biol*. 1990; 270: 83-93.
42. Fernando H.A, Zibellini J, Harris R.A, et al. "Effect of Ramadan Fasting on Weight and Body Composition in Healthy Non-Athlete Adults: A Systematic Review and Meta-Analysis." *Nutrients*. 2019; 11:478.
43. Abdullah K, AL-Habori M, Al-Eryani E. "Ramadan Intermittent Fasting Affects Adipokines and Leptin/Adiponectin Ratio in Type 2 Diabetes Mellitus and Their First-Degree Relatives." *Bio Med Res Int*. 2020; 1281192
44. BaHammam A.S, Almeneessier A.S. "Recent Evidence on the Impact of Ramadan Diurnal Intermittent Fasting, Mealtime, and Circadian Rhythm on Cardiometabolic Risk: A Review." *Front Nutr*. 2020;7: 28
45. Stern L, Iqbal N, Seshadri P, et al. "The effects of low-carbohydrate versus conventional weight-loss diets in severely obese adults: one-year follow-up of a randomized trial." *Ann Intern Med*. 2004; 140: 778-85.
46. Petrisko M, Kloss R, Bradley P, et al. "Biochemical, Anthropometric, and Physiological Responses to Carbohydrate-Restricted Diets Versus a Low Fat Diet in Obese Adults: A Randomized Crossover Trial." *J Med Food*. 2020; 23: 206-14.
47. Mirza N.M, Palmer M.G, Sinclair K.B, et al. "Effects of a low glycemic load or a low-fat dietary intervention on body weight in obese Hispanic American children and adolescents: a randomized controlled trial." *Am J Clin Nutr*. 2013; 97: 276-85.
48. Voegtlin W.L. *Stone Age Diet*. Vantage Press. New York. 1975.
49. Eaton S.B, Eaton S.B 3rd, Konner M.J. "Palaeolithic nutrition revisited: a twelve year retrospective on its nature and implications." *Eur J Clin Nutr*. 2013; 368: 1279-90.
50. Cordain L, Eaton SB, Miller JB, et al. "The paradoxical nature of hunter-gatherer diets meat-based, yet non-atherogenic." *Eur J Clin Nutr*. 2002; 56: 542-52.
51. Cordain L, Miller J.B, Eaton S.B, et al. "Macronutrient estimation in hunter-gatherer diet." *Am J Clin Nutr*. 2000: 72: 1589-92.
52. Estruch R, Ros E, Salas-Salvadó JS, et al. "Primary prevention of cardiovascular disease with a Mediterranean diet supplemented with extra-virgin oil and nuts." *N Engl J Med*. 2013; 378: e34.
53. Mitrou P.N, Kipnis V, Thiébaut A.C, et al. "Mediterranean dietary pattern and prediction of all-cause mortality in a US population:

results from the NIH-AARP Diet and Health Study." *Arch Intern Med.* 2007; 167: 2461-8.
54. Vásquez-Builes S, Paulina Jaramillo-Echeverri P, Montoya-Quinchia L. et al. "Dieta cetogénica como tratamiento de la epilepsia refractaria durante la infancia: revisión práctica de la literatura." .*RevMex Neuroc.*2019; 20: 14-20.
55. Verrotti A, Iapadre G, Di Francesco L, et al. "Diet in the Treatment of Epilepsy: What We Know So Far" *Nutrients*. 2020; 12: 2645
56. Yudlko M, Daikhin Y, Horyn O, et al. "Ketosis and brain handling of glutamate, glutamine and GABA." *Epilepsia*. 2008; 49: 73-5.
57. Appel L.J, Moore T.J, Obarzanek E, et al. "A clinical trial of the effects of dietary patterns on blood pressure. DASH Collaborative Research Group." *N Engl J Med*. 1997; 336: 1117-24.
58. Ornish D, Scherwitz L.W, Billings J.H, et al. "Intensive lifestyle changes for reversal of coronary heart disease." *JAMA* 1998; 280: 2001-7
59. Ding M, Rexrode K.M. "A Review of Lipidomics of Cardiovascular Disease Highlights the Importance of Isolating Lipoproteins." *Metabolites*. 2020; 10: 163.
60. Simons LA, Simon S.J, Friedlander Y et al. "Cholesterol and other lipids predict coronary heart disease and ischaemic stroke in the elderly, but only in those below 70 years." *Atherosclerosis*. 2001; 159: 201.
61. Knopp R.H, Retzlaff B.M. "Saturated fat prevents coronary artery disease? An American paradox." *Am J Clin Nutr*. 2004; 80: 1102-3.
62. Petousis-Harris H. "Saturated fat has been unfairly demonised: yes." *J Prim Health Care*. 2011; 3: 317-9.
63. Skeaff C.M, Jackson R. "Saturated fat has been unfairly demonised: no." *J Prim Health Care*. 2011; 3: 320-21.
64. Ravnskov U. "The questionable role of saturated and polyunsaturated fatty acids in cardiovascular disease." *J Clin Epidemiol.*1998; 51: 443-60.
65. Virtanen J.K. "Randomized trials of replacing saturated fatty acids with n-6 polyunsaturated fatty acids in coronary heart disease prevention: Not the gold standard? Prostaglandins Leukot Essential Fatty Acids." 2018; 133: 8-15.
66. Siri-Tarino P.W., Sun Q., Hu F.B., et al. "Meta-analysis of prospective cohort studies evaluating the association of saturated fat with cardiovascular disease." *Am J Clin Nut.*2010; 91: 535-46.

67. Siri-Tarino P.W., Sun Q., Hu F.B., et al. "Saturated fat, carbohydrate and cardiovascular disease." *Am J Clin Nutr.* 2010; 91: 502-9
68. Astrup A, Dyerberg J, Elwood P, et al. "The role of reducing intakes of saturated fat in the prevention of cardiovascular disease: where does the evidence stand in 2010?" *Am J Clin Nutr.* 2011: 93: 684-8.
69. Rychter A.M, Ratajczak A.E, Zawada A, et al. "Non-Systematic Review of Diet and Nutritional Risk Factors of Cardiovascular Disease in Obesity." *Nutrients*. 2020; 12: 814.
70. Mozaffarian D, Katan M.B, Ascherio A, et al. "Trans Fatty Acids and Cardiovascular Disease." *N Engl J Med.* 2006; 354: 1601-13.
71. Bhardwaj S, Passi S.J, Misra A. "Overview of trans fatty acids: biochemistry and health effects." *Diabetes Metab Syndr.* 2011; 5:161-64.
72. Lopez-Garcia E, Schulze M.B, Meigs J.B, et al. "Consumption of *Trans* Fatty Acids Is Related to Plasma Biomarkers of Inflammation and Endothelial Dysfunction." *J Nutr.* 2005; 135: 562-6.
73. Mozaffarian D, Katan M.B, Ascherio A, et al. "Trans Fatty Acids and Cardiovascular Disease." *N Engl J Med.*2008; 354: 1601-13.
74. Koletzko B, Muller J. "Cis- and trans-isomeric fatty acids in plasma lipids of newborn infants and their mothers." *Biol Neonate.* 1990; 57: 172-8.
75. Peterson G, Aguilar D, Especheh M, y col. "Ácidos grasos trans en alimentos consumidos habitualmente por los jóvenes en Argentina." *Arch Argent Pediatr.* 2004; 102:102-9.
76. Sandra L, Elias S.I, "Infant plasma *trans*, n−6, and n−3 fatty acids and conjugated linoleic acids are related to maternal plasma fatty acids, length of gestation, and birth weight and length." *Am J Clin Nutr.* 2001; 73: 807-14.
77. Upritard J.E, Zeelenberg M.J, Huizinga H, et al. "Modern fat technology: what is the potential for heart health?" *Proc Nutr Soc.* 2005; 64: 379-86.
78. Tarrago-Trani M.T, Phillips K.M, Lemar L.E, et al. "New and existing oils and fats used in products with reduced trans-fatty acid content." *J Am Diet Assoc.*2006; 106: 867-80.
79. Shanahan C, Shanahan L. *Deep Nutrition.* Flatiron Books. New York. 2017.

80. Lombard C.B. "What is the role of food in preventing depression and improving mood, performance and cognitive function?" *Med J Aust.* 2000; 173 Suppl: S104-5.
81. Nemets B, Stahl Z, Belmaker R.H. "Addition of omega-3 fatty acid to maintenance medication treatment for recurrent unipolar depressive disorder." *Am J Psychiatry.* 2002; 159: 477-9
82. Mozafforiam D, Wu.J.H. "(n-3) Fatty Acids and Cardiovascular Health: Are Effects of EPA and DHA Shared or Complementary?" *J Nutr.* 2012; 142:614S-25S.
83. Garman J, Mulroney S, Manigrasso M, et al. "Omega-3 fatty acid rich diet prevents diabetic renal disease." *Am J Physiol Renal Physiol.* 2009; 296:306-16
84. Kelly G. "Inulin-type prebiotic. A Review: part 1." *Altern Med Rev.* 2008; 13: 315-29.
85. Astó E, Méndez I, Rodríguez-Prado M, et al. "Effect of the Degree of Polymerization of Fructans on Ex Vivo Fermented Human Gut Microbiome." *Nutrients.* 2019; 11: 1293.
86. Valenzuela A, Maiz AG. "El rol de la fibra en la alimentación enteral." *Rev Chil Nutr.* 2006; 33: 342-56
87. Whisner C.M, Weaver C.M. "Galacto-oligosaccharides: Probiotic effect on calcium absorption and bone health." En: *Nutritional Influences on Bone Health.* Springer-Verlag. London. 2013: 315-23.
88. Quintero-García M, Gutiérrez-Cortez E, Rojas-Molina A, et al. "Calcium Bioavailability of *Opuntia ficus-indica* Cladodes in an Ovariectomized Rat Model of Postmenopausal Bone Loss." *Nutrients.*2020; 12: 1431
89. Jenkins D.J.A, Kendall S.W.C, Augustin L.S.A, et al. "Glycemic index: overview of implications in health and disease." *Am J Clin Nutr.* 2002; 76: 2665-735
90. Steen E, Terry B.M, Rivera E.J, et al. "Impaired insulin and insulin-like growth factor expression and signaling mechanisms in Alzheimer's disease is this type 3 diabetes?" *J Alzheimers Dis.* 2005; 7: 63-80.
91. Nam K.H, An S.Y, Joo Y.S, et al. "Carbohydrate-Rich Diet Is Associated with Increased Risk of Incident Chronic Kidney Disease in Non-Diabetic Subjects." *J Clin Med.* 2019; 8: 793.
92. Foster-Powell, Holt S.H.A, Brand-Miller J.C." International table of glycemic index and glycemic load values: 2002." *Am J Clin Nutr.* 2002; 76: 5–56

93. Fiona S, Atkinson R.D, Kaye Foster-Powell R.D, et al. "International Tables of Glycemic Index and Glycemic Load Values." *Diabetes Care*. 2008; 31: 2261-63.
94. Suez J, Korem T, Zeevi D, et al. "Artificial sweeteners induce glucose intolerance by altering the gut microbiota." *Nature*. 2014. 514: 181-6.
95. Blundell J.E, Hill A.J. "Paradoxical effects of an intense sweetener (aspartame) on appetite." *Lancet*.1986; 1: 1092-3.
96. Jing M.A, Bellon M, Wishart J, et al. "Effect of the artificial sweetener, sucralose, on gastric emptying and incretin hormone release in healthy subjects." *Am J PhysiolGastrointest Liver Physiol*. 2009; 296: 735-9.
97. Ray J, Kumar S, Laor D et al. "Effects of *Stevia Rebaudiana* on Glucose Homeostasis, Blood Pressure and Inflammation: A Critical Review of Past and Current Research Evidence." *Int J Clin Res Trials*. 2020; 5: 142-50.
98. Rizwan F, Ur Rashid H, Yesmine, S, et al. "Preliminary analysis of the effect of Stevia (*Stevia rebaudiana*) in patients with chronic kidney disease (stage I to stage III)." *Contemp Clin Trials Commun*. 2018; 12: 17–25.
99. Braakhuis A. "Evidence on the Health Benefits of Supplemental Propolis." *Nutrients*. 2019; 11: 2705.
100. Cornara L, Biagi M, Xiao J, et al. "Therapeutic properties of bioactive compounds from different honeybee products." *Front Pharmacol*. 2017; 8: 412.
101. Alkis H, Kuzhan A, Dirier A, et al. "Neuroprotective effects of propolis and caffeic acid phenethyl ester (CAPE) on the radiation-injured brain tissue (Neuroprotective effects of propolis and CAPE)." *Int J Radiat Res*. 2015; 13: 297-303.
102. Tolba M.F, Esmat A, Al-Abd A.M, et al. "Caffeic acid phenethyl ester synergistically enhances docetaxel and paclitaxel cytotoxicity in prostate cancer cell." *IOUBMLife*. 2013; 65: 716-29.
103. Haddadin M, Nazer I, Jamal S, et al. "Effect of propolis on two bacterial species with probiotic potential. Pak J Nutr. 2008; 7: 391–94.
104. Silveira M.A.D, Teles F, Berretta A.A, et al. "Effects of Brazilian green propolis on proteinuria and renal function in patients with chronic kidney disease: a randomized, double-blind, placebo-controlled trial." *BMC Nephrol*. 2019; 20: 140.

105. Li Y.J, Lin J.L, Yang C.W, et al. "Acute renal failure induced by a Brazilian variety of propolis." *Am J Kidney Dis*. 2005; 46: e125–e129.
106. Cao G, Ying P, Yan B, et al. "Pharmacokinetics, safety, and tolerability of single and multiple-doses of pinocembrin injection administered intravenously in healthy subjects." *J Ethnopharmacol.* 2015; 168: 31–6.
107. Cao X.P, Chen Y.F, Zhang J.L, et al. "Mechanisms underlying the wound healing potential of propolis based on its in vitro antioxidant activity." *Phytomed*. 2017; 34: 76–84.
108. Moncada S, Higgs A. "The L-Arginine-Nitric Oxide Pathway." *N Engl J Med.* 1993; 329: 2002-12.
109. National Academy of Sciences. Institute of Medicine.Food and Nutrition Board. Dietary Reference Intakes for Energy, Carbohydrate, Fibre, Fat, Fatty Acids, Cholesterol, Protein and Amino Acids Macronutrients. 2005.
110. Boschmann M, Steiniger J, Franke G, et al. "Water drinking induces thermogenesis through osmosensitive mechanisms."*J Clin Endocrinol Metab*. 2007; 92: 3334-7.
111. Davy B.M, Dennis E.A, Dengo A.L, et al. "Water consumption reduces energy intake at a breakfast meal in obese older adults."*J Am Diet Assoc*. 2008; 108:1236-9.
109. Van Walleghen E.L, Orr J.S, Gentile C.L, et al. "Pre-meal water consumption reduces meal energy intake in older but not younger subjects." *Obesity* (Silver Spring). 2007; 15: 93-9.
110. Dennis E.A, Dengo A.L, Comber D.L, et al. "Water consumption increases weight loss during a hypocaloric diet intervention in middle-aged and older adults." *Obesity* (Silver Spring). 2010; 18: 300-7.
111. Thornton SN. "Increased Hydration Can Be Associated with Weight Loss." *Front Nutr*. 2016; 3: 18.
112. Harper C. "The neuropathology of alcohol-related brain damage." *Alcohol.* 2009; 44: 136-40.
113. Oscar-Berman M, Marinkovic K. "Alcohol: effects on neurobehavioural functions and the brain." *Neuropsychol Rev.* 2007; 17: 239-57.
114. Fowler A.K, Hewetson A, Agrawal R.G, et al. "Alcohol-induced One-carbon Metabolism Impairment Promotes Dysfunction of DNA Base Excision Repair in Adult Brain." *J Biol Chem.* 2012; 287: 43533-42.

115. Auger C, Alhasawi A, Contavadoo M, et al. "Dysfunctional mitochondrial bioenergetics and the pathogenesis of hepatic disorders." *Front Cell Dev Biol*. 2015; 3: 40.
116. Erdozain A.M, Morentin B, Bedford L, et al. "Alcohol-Related Brain Damage in Humans." *PLoS ONE*. 2014; 9: e93586.
117. González-Reimers E, Santolaria-Fernández F, Martín-González M.C, et al. "Alcoholism: A systemic proinflammatory condition." *World J Gastroenterol*. 2014; 20:14660-71.
118. Queipo-Ortuño M.I, Boto-Ordóñez M, Murri M, et al. "Influence of red wine polyphenols and ethanol on the gut microbiota ecology and biochemical biomarkers." *Am J Clin Nutr*. 2012; 95:1323-34.
119. Hervert-Hernandez D, GoñiI. "Dietary polyphenols and human gut microbiota: a review." *Food Rev Int*. 2011; 27: 154–69.
120. Rogne T, Tielemans MJ, Chong M.F, et al. "Associations of Maternal Vitamin B12 Concentration in Pregnancy With the Risks of Preterm Birth and Low Birth Weight: A Systematic Review and Meta-Analysis of Individual Participant Data." *Am J Epidemiol*. 2017; 185: 212-23.
121. Shargorodsky M, Debby O, Matas Z, et al. "Effect of long-term treatment with antioxidants (vitamin C, vitamin E, coenzyme Q10 and selenium) on arterial compliance, humoral factors and inflammatory markers in patients with multiple cardiovascular risk factors." *NutrMetab*.2010; 7: 5
122. Hong J.Y, Lee C.Y, Lee M.G, et al. "Effects of dietary antioxidant vitamins on lung functions according to gender and smoking status in Korea: a population-based cross-sectional study." *Brit Med J* Open. 2018; 8: e 020656.
123. Kevany J, Jessop W, Goldsmith A, et al. "The effect of smoking on ascorbic acid and serum cholesterol in adult males." *Ir J Med Sci*. 1975; 144: 474.
124. Pelletier O. "Smoking and Vitamin C Levels In Humans." *Amer J Clin Nutr*. 1968; 21:1259-67.
125. Hemilä H. "Vitamin C supplementation and common cold symptoms: problems with inaccurate reviews." *Nutrition*. 1996; 12: 804-9.
126. Shargorodsky M, Debby O, Matas Z, et al. "Effect of long-term treatment with antioxidants (vitamin C, vitamin E, coenzyme Q10 and selenium) on arterial compliance, humoral factors and inflammatory markers in patients with multiple cardiovascular risk factors." *Nutr Metab*. 2010; 7: 55.

127. Hemilä H. "Vitamin C and common cold-induced asthma: a systematic review and statistical analysis." *Allergy, Asthma & Clin Immunol.* 2013; **9**: 46.
128. Giovannucci E, Liu Y, Rimm E.B, et al. "Prospective study of predictors of vitamin D status and cancer incidence and mortality in men." *J Natl Cancer Inst*. 2006; 98: 451-9.
129. González Pardo V, Boland R, Russo de Boland A. "Vitamina D y cáncer: Acción antineoplásica de la 1α,25$(OH)_2$-Vitamina D_3" *Medicina* (Buenos Aires). 2012; 72: 143-9.
130. Ding Ch, Wilding J.P.H, Bing, Ch. "1,25-dihydroxy vitamin D_3 Protects against Macrophage-Induced Activation of NFκB and MAPK Signalling and Chemokine Release in Human Adipocytes." *PLoSOne*. 2013; 8: e61707.
131. Ginanjar E, Sumariyono, Setiati S, et al. "VitaminD and autoimmune disease."*Acta Med Indones* .2007; 39: 133-41.
132. Mathieu C, Badenhoop K. "Vitamin D and type 1 diabetes mellitus: state of the art." *Trends Endocrinol Metab.* 2005;16: 261-6.
133. Martineau A.R, Jolliffe D.A, Hooper R.L, et al. "Vitamin D supplementation to prevent acute respiratory tract infections: systematic review and meta-analysis of individual participant data." *BMJ.* 2017; 356: i6583.
134. Wortsman J, Matsuoka L.Y, Chen T.C, et al. "Decreased bioavailability of vitamin D in obesity." *Am J Clin Nutr*. 2000; 72: 690-3.
135. Rodríguez-Rodríguez E, Aparicio Vizuete A, Sánchez-Rodríguez P, et al. "Deficiencia en vitamina D de la población española. Importancia del huevo en la mejora nutricional [Vitamin D deficiency in Spanish population. Importance of egg on nutritional improvement]." *Nutr Hosp*. 2019; 36: 3-7.
136. McNamara D.J. "The Fifty Year Rehabilitation of the Egg." *Nutrients*. 2015; 7: 8716-22.
137. Réhault-Godbert S, Guyot N, Nys Y. "The Golden Egg: Nutritional Value, Bioactivities, and Emerging Benefits for Human Health." *Nutrients.* 2019; 11: 684.
138. Wang M.X, Wong C.H, Kim J.E."Impact of whole egg intake on blood pressure, lipids and lipoproteins in middle-aged and older population: A systematic review and meta-analysis of randomized controlled trials."*Nutr Metab Cardiovasc Dis*. 2019; 29: 653-64.
139. Zhang X, Lv M, Luo X, et al. "Egg consumption and health outcomes: a global evidence mapping based on an overview of systematic reviews." *Ann Transl Med.* 2020; 8: 1343.

140. Lee Y, Han C.Y, Bae M, et al.”Egg phospholipids exert an inhibitory effect on intestinal cholesterol absorption in mice.“ *Nutr Res Pract*. 2019; 13: 295-301.
141. Escudero P. “Las vitaminas. (Segunda Parte).” En: *Alimentación*. 109. Librería Hachette S.A. Buenos Aires. 1934.
142. Weir M.R, Dworkin L.D. “Antihypertensive drugs, dietary salt, and renal protection: how low should you go and with which therapy?” *Am J Kidney Dis*. 1998; 32: 1-22.
143. WHO issues new guidance on dietary salt and potassium. 2013.
144. Yamaguchi S, Ninomiya K. “Umami and Food Palatability.” *J Nutr*. 2000; 130: 921S–26S.
145. Yamamoto S, Tomoe M, Toyama K, et al. “¿Puede mejorar la salud de los adultos mayores con suplementos de glutamato monosódico?” *Am J Clin Nutr*. 2009; 90: 844S-9S.
146. Voyer Luis E., Medio Interno. “Fisiología, patología y tratamiento de los líquidos orgánicos.” Pg 47. *Ed. Journal*. Buenos Aires. 2017.
147. Alkhaldy A, Edwards C.A, Combet E. “The urinary phenolic acid profile varies between younger and older adults after a polyphenol-rich meal despite limited differences in in vitro colonic catabolism.” *Eur J Nutr*. 2019; 58: 1095-111.
148. Vauzour D. “Dietary polyphenols as modulators of brain functions: biological actions and molecular mechanisms underpinning their beneficial effects.” *Oxid Med Cell Longev*. 2012; 2012: 914273.
149. Pandareesh M.D, Mythri R.B, Srinivas Bharath M.M. “Bioavailability of dietary polyphenols: Factors contributing to their clinical application in CNS diseases.” *Neurochem Int*. 2015; 89: 198-208.
150. Wong H.L, Wu X.Y, Bendayan R. “Nanotechnological advances for the delivery of CNS therapeutics.” *Adv Drug Deliv Rev*. 2012; 64: 686-700.
151. Saeedi M, Eslamifar M, Khezri K, et al. “Applications of nanotechnology in drug delivery to the central nervous system.” *Biomed Pharmacother*. 2019; 111: 666-75.
152. Liu R, Wu C, Zhou D, et al. “Pinocembrin protects against β-amyloid-induced toxicity in neurons through inhibiting receptor for advanced glycation end products (RAGE)-independent signaling pathways and regulating mitochondrion-mediated apoptosis.” B.M.C Med. 2012; 10, 105.
153. Bondonno C.P, Croft K.D, Hodgson J.M. “Dietary Nitrate, Nitric Oxide, and Cardiovascular Health.” *Crit Rev Food Sci Nutr*. 2016; 56: 2036-52.

154. Brayan Moreno C., Karen Soto O., Daniel González R. "El consumo de nitrato y su potencial efectobenéfico. Nitrate consumption and potential beneficial effect on cardiovascular health." *Rev Chi Nutr.* 2015; 42 (2).
155. Williams M.J.A, Sutherland W.H.F, McCormick M.P. et al. "Impaired endothelial function following a meal rich in used cooking fat." *J Am Coll Cardiol.* 1999; 33: 1050–55.
126. Shargorodsky M, Debby O, Matas Z, et al. "Effect of long-term treatment with antioxidants (vitamin C, vitamin E, coenzyme Q10 and selenium) on arterial compliance, humoral factors and inflammatory markers in patients with multiple cardiovascular risk factors." *Nutr Metab.* 2010; 7: 55.
127. Hemilä H. "Vitamin C and common cold-induced asthma: a systematic review and statistical analysis." *Allergy, Asthma & Clin Immunol.* 2013; 9: 46.
128. Giovannucci E, Liu Y, Rimm E.B, et al. "Prospective study of predictors of vitamin D status and cancer incidence and mortality in men." *J Natl Cancer Inst.* 2006; 98: 451-9.
129. González Pardo V, Boland R, Russo de Boland A. "Vitamina D y cáncer: Acción antineoplásica de la $1\alpha,25(OH)_2$-Vitamina D_3" *Medicina* (Buenos Aires). 2012; 72: 143-9.
130. Ding Ch, Wilding J.P.H, Bing, Ch. "1,25-dihydroxy vitamin D_3 Protects against Macrophage-Induced Activation of NFκB and MAPK Signalling and Chemokine Release in Human Adipocytes." *PLoSOne.* 2013; 8: e61707.
131. Ginanjar E, Sumariyono, Setiati S, et al. "VitaminD and autoimmune disease."*Acta Med Indones* .2007; 39: 133-41.
132. Mathieu C, Badenhoop K. "Vitamin D and type 1 diabetes mellitus: state of the art." *Trends Endocrinol Metab.* 2005;16: 261-6.
157. Sikora E. Cieślik E, Topolska K."The sources of natural antioxidants." Acta Sci Pol. Technol. Aliment. 2008; 7: 5-17.
158. Shanahan C, Shanahan L. "How your doctor can tell if you have french-fried arteries: erectile dysfunction and endothelial function." In: *Deep Nutrition.* Chapter 7, 144-145. Flatiron Books Edition. 2017. New York.
159. Conzatti A, Telles da Silva Fróes F.C, Schweigert PerryI.D, y col. "Evidencias clínicas y moleculares del consumo de brócoli, glucorafanina y sulforafano en humanos." *Nutr Hosp.* 2015; 31: 7685.
160. Soliman M.M, Nassan M.A, Aldhahrani A, et al. "Molecular and Histopathological Study on the Ameliorative Impacts of Petroselinum

Crispum and Apium Graveolens against Experimental Hyperuricemia." *Sci Rep*. 2020; 10: 9512.
161. Siegel S. *Pleiotropic effect of garlic*. Wien Med Wochensschr. 1999; 149: 217-24.
162. Bayan L, Kouliband P.H, Gorji A. "Garlic: Review of potential therapeutic effects." *Avicena J Phytomed*. 2014; 4: 1-14.
163. Biró A, Markovics A, Fazekas M.É, et al. "Allithiamine Alleviates Hyperglycaemia-Induced Endothelial Dysfunction." *Nutrients*. 2020; 12:1690.
164. Fontana G, Bruno M, Notarbarolo N, et al."Cytotoxicity of oleanolic and ursolic acid derivatives toward hepatocellular carcinoma and evaluation of NF-κB involvement." *Biolog Chem*. 2019; 90:103054.
165. Wang Y.S, Li G.L, Zhu S.B, et al. "A Self-assembled Nanoparticle Platform Based on AmphiphilicOleanolic Acid Polyprodrug for Cancer Therapy." *Chin J Polym Sci.* 2020; 38: 819-29.
166. Franke A.A, Cooney R.V, Henning S.M, et al. "Bioavailability and antioxidant effects of orange juice components in humans." *J Agric Food Chem*. 2005; 53: 5170-78.
167. Sanchez-Moreno C, Cano M.P, De Ancos B, et al. "Effect of orange juice intake on vitamin C concentrations and biomarkers of antioxidant status in humans." *Am J Clin Nutr*. 2003; 78: 454-60.
168. Deng G.F, Lin X, Xu X.R, et al. "Antioxidant capacities and total phenolic contents of 56 vegetables." *J Funct Foods.* 2013; 5: 26066.
169. Singh B, Singh J.P, Kaur A, et al. "Bioactive compounds in banana and their associated health benefits. A review." *Food Chem*. 2016; 206: 1-11.
170. Powthong P, Jantrapanukorn B, Suntornthiticharoen P, et al. "Study of prebiotic properties of selected banana species in Thailand." *Food Sci Technol*. 2020; 57: 2490-500.
171. Santana L.F, Inada A.C, Espirito Santo B.L.S.D, et al. "Nutraceutical Potential of *Carica papaya* in Metabolic Syndrome." *Nutrients*. 2019; 11: 1608.
172. Vij T, Prashar Y. "A review on medicinal properties of *Carica papaya* Linn." *Asian Pac J Trop Dis*. 2015; 5: 1-6.
173. Shah K.A, Patel M.B, Patel R.J, et al. "Mangifera indica (mango)." *Pharmacogn Rev*. 2010; 4: 42-8.
174. Lu S.C. "Glutathione synthesis." *Biochim Biophys Acta*. 2013; 1830: 3143-53.

175. Vivero S.A, Valenzuela B.R, Valenzuela B.A, et al. "Palta: compuestos bioactivos y sus potenciales beneficios en salud." *Rev Chil Nutr*. 2019; 46.
176. Reddy M, Moodley R, Jonnalagadda S.B. "Fatty acid profile and elemental content of avocado (Persea americana Mill) oil-effect of extraction methods." *J Environ Sci Health B* 2012; 47: 529-37.
177. Guzmán-Rodríguez J.J, López-Gómez R, Salgado-Garciglia R, et al. "The defensin from avocado (Persea americana var. drymifolia) PaDef induces apoptosis in the human breast cancer cell line MCF-7." *Biomed Pharmacother*. 2016; 82: 620-7.
178. Aviram M, Rosenblat M, Gaitini D, et al. "Pomegranate juice consumption for 3 years by patients with carotid artery stenosis reduces common carotid intima-media thickness, blood pressure and LDL oxidation." *Clin Nutr*. 2004; 23: 423-33.
179. Mills E.N, Mackie A.R. "The impact of processing on allergenicity of food." *Curr Opin Allergy Clin Immunol*. 2008; 8: 249-53.
180. Vitale A.A, Bernatene E.A, Pomilio A.B. "Carotenoides en quimioprevención: Licopenos." *Acta Bioquim Clin Latinoam*. 2010;44: 195-8.
181. Stahl W. Heinrich U, Wiseman S, et al. "Dietary tomato paste protects against ultraviolet light-induced erythema in humans." *J Nutr*. 2001; 131: 1449-51.
182. Koppmann M. "El chocolate y sus misterios." *Ciencia Hoy*. 2014; 24: 61-4.
183. Ferreira H.S, dos Santos A.F., et al. "Effects of dietary coconut oil on the biochemical and anthropometric profiles of women presenting abdominal obesity." *Lipids*.2009; 44: 593-601.
184. Oliveira-de-Lira L, Santos E.M.C, de Souza R.F, et al. "Supplementation-Dependent Effects of Vegetable Oils with Varying Fatty Acid Compositions on Anthropometric and Biochemical Parameters in Obese Women." *Nutrients*. 2018; 10: 932.
185. Vasconcelos L.H.C, Silva M.C.C, Costa A.C, et al. "Virgin Coconut Oil Supplementation Prevents Airway Hyperreactivity of Guinea Pigs with Chronic Allergic Lung Inflammation by Antioxidant Mechanism." *Oxid Med Cell Longev*. 2020; 2020: 5148-503.
186. Trowell HC. "The development of the concept of dietary fibre in human nutrition." *Am J Clin Nutr*. 1978; 31: 53-111.
187. Cummings J.H, Engineer A. "Denis Burkitt and the origins of the dietary fibre hypothesis." *Nutr Res Rev*. 2018; 31: 1-15.

188. Burkitt D.P, Walker A.R.P, Painter J.N.S. "Effect of dietary fibre stools and transit- times, and its role in the causation of disease." *Lancet* 1972; 2:1408-14.
189. Burkitt D.P, Walker A.R.P, Painter J.N.S. "Dietary fiber and disease." *J Am MedAssoc*. 1974; 229: 1068-74.
190. Strte L.L. "Diverticulosis y fibra dietética." *Gastroenterology*. 2012; 142: 205-10.
191. Veronese N, Solmi M, Caruso MG, e.t al. "Dietary fibre and health outcomes: an umbrella review of systematic reviews and meta-analyses." *Am J Clin Nutr*. 2018; 107: 436-44.
156. Dimina L, Mariotti F. "The Postprandial Appearance of Features of Cardiometabolic Risk: Acute Induction and Prevention by Nutrients and Other Dietary Substances." *Nutrients*. 2019; 11: 1963.
192. Almeida-Alvarado S.L, Aguilar-López T, Hervert-Hernández D. "La fibra y sus beneficios a la salud" *An Venez Nutr*. 2014; 27 (1).
193. Paulo A.Z, Amancio O.M.S., de Morais M.B., et al. "Low-dietary fibre intake as a risk factor for recurrent abdominal pain in children." *Europ J Clinl Nutr*. 2006; 60: 823-7.
194. Puértolas-Balint F, Schroeder B.O. 2 "Does an Apple a Day Also Keep the Microbes Away? The Interplay Between Diet, Microbiota and Host Defense Peptides at the Intestinal Mucosal Barrier." *Front Immunol*. 2020; 11: 1164.
195. Yazdi F.G, Soleimanian-Zad S, van den Worm E, et al. "Turmeric Extract: Potential Use as a Prebiotic and Anti-Inflammatory Compound?" *Plant Foods Hum Nutr*. 2019; 74: 293-99.
196. Trowell H.C. "Dietary fibre, ischaemic heart disease and diabetes mellitus." *Proc. Nutr. Soc*. 1973; 32: 151-7.
197. Burri L, Johnsen L. "Krill Products: An Overview of Animal Studies." *Nutrients* 2015; *7:* 3300-21.
198. Herron K.L, Lofgren I.E, Sharman M.J, et al. "High intake of cholesterol results in less atherogenic low-density lipoprotein particles in men and women independent of response classification." *Metabolism*. 2004; 53: 823-30.
199. Fernandez M.L. "Rethinking dietary cholesterol." *Curr Opin Clin Nutr Metab Care*.2012; 15: 117-21.
200. Gonnzález Matute R, Figlas N.D, Postemsky P. et al. "Hongos comestibles y medicinales." *Ciencia Hoy*. 2011; 20: 9-15.
201. Cano-Estrad A, Romero-Bautista L. "Valor económico, nutricional y medicinal de hongos comestibles silvestres." *Rev Chil Nutr*. 2016; 43.

202. Kwaifa I.K, Bahari H, Yong Y.K, et al. "Endothelial Dysfunction in Obesity-Induced Inflammation: Molecular Mechanisms and Clinical Implications." Biomolecules. 2020 13; 10: 291.
203. Li Y, Liu H, Zhang L, et al. "Maternal Dietary Fibre Composition during Gestation Induces Changes in Offspring Antioxidative Capacity, Inflammatory Response, and Gut Microbiota in a Sow Model." *Int J Mol Sci*. 2019; 21: 31.
204. Rosa F.T, Freitas E.C, Deminice R et al. "Oxidative stress and inflammation in obesity after taurine supplementation: a double-blind, placebo-controlled study." *Eur J Nut.*2014; 53: 823–30.
205. Teff K.L, Elliott S.S, Tschöp M, et al. "Dietary fructose reduces circulating insulin and leptin, attenuates postprandial suppression of ghrelin, and increases triglycerides in women." *J Clin Endocrinol Metab*. 2004; 89: 2963-72.
206. Klöting N, Fasshauer M, Dietrich A, et al. "Insulin sensitive obesity." *Am J Physiol Endocrinol Metab*. 2010; 299: E506-15.
207. Matsuzawa Y. "Establishment of a concept of visceral fat syndrome and discovery of adiponectin." *Proc Jpn Acad Ser B Phys Biol Sci*. 2010; 86: 131-41.
208. Marchetti P, Lupi R, Del Guerra S, et al. "The beta-cell in human type 2 diabetes." *Adv Exp Med Biol*. 2010; 654: 501-14.
209. Guerrero-Romero F, Rodríguez Moran M. "Metabolically obese normal-weight children." *World J Clin Pediatr*. 2012; 1: 37-9.
210. Ruderman N.B, Schneider S.H, Berchtold P. "The 'metabolically-obese' normal-weight individual." *Am J Clin Nutr*. 1981; 34:1617-21.
211. Kelisadi R, Hashemipour M, Sarrafzadegan N., et al. "Effects of a lifestyle modification trial among phenotypically obese metabolically normal and phenotypically obese metabolically abnormal adolescents in comparison with phenotypically normal metabolically obese adolescents" *Matern Child Nutr*. 2010; 6: 275–86.
212. de Hollander E, Bemelmans WJE, Boshuizen HC, et al. "The association between waist circumference and risk of mortality considering body mass index in 65- to 74-year-olds: a meta-analysis of 29 cohorts involving more than 58 000 elderly persons."*Int J Epidemiol*. 2012; 41: 805-17.
213. Ross R, Neeland I.J, Yamashita S., et al. "Waist circumference as a vital sign in clinical practice: a Consensus Statement from the IAS and ICCR Working Group on Visceral Obesity." *Nat Rev Endocrinol*. 2020; 16: 177-89.

214. Declèves A.E, Sharma K. "Obesity and kidney disease: differential effects of obesity on adipose tissue and kidney inflammation and fibrosis." *Curr Opin Nephrol Hypertens*. 2015; 24: 28-36.
215. Shin E, Koo J.S. "The Role of Adipokines and Bone Marrow Adipocytes in Breast Cancer Bone Metastasis." *Int J Mol Sci*. 2020; 21: 4967.
216. Blüher M, Mantzoros C.S. "From leptin to other adipokines in health anddisease: facts and expectations at the beginning of the 21st century." *Metabolism*. 2015; 64: 131-45.
217. Adamczak M, Wiecek A. "The adipose tissue as an endocrine organ." *Semin Nephro*l. 2013; 33: 2-13.
218. Ford E, Giles W.A. "A comparison of the prevalence of the metabolic syndrome using two proposed definitions." *Diabetes Care*. 2003; 26: 575-81.
219. NCEP: National Cholesterol Education Program. Adult Treatment. JAMA. 2010; 299: E506-15.
220. Alen R.W, Schwartzman E, Baker W.L, et al. "Cinnamon use in type 2 diabetes. An update systemic review and metanalysis." *Ann Fam Med*. 2013; 115: 452-9.
221. Golomb B.A, Evans M.A. "Statin adverse effects: a review of the literature and evidence for a mitochondrial mechanism." *Am J Cardiovasc Drugs*. 2008; 8: 373-418.
222. Acosta A.H, Escalona M, Maiz A, y col. "Determinación del índice de resistencia insulinica mediante HOMA en una población de la región metropolitana de Chile." *Rev Med Chile*. 2002; 130: 1227-31.
223. Garmendia M.L, Lera L, Sánchez H, y col. "Valores normativos de resistencia a la insulina mediante HOMA-IR en adultos mayores de Santiago Chile." *Rev Med Chile*. 2009; 137: 1409-16.
224. Xu Y, Guo W, Zhang CH. "Herbal Medicine in the Treatment of Non-Alcoholic Fatty Liver Diseases-Efficacy, Action Mechanism and Clinical Application Pharmacol." 2020; 12 May.
225. Díaz-Rizzolo D, Kostov B, López Siles M, et al. "Healthy dietary pattern and their corresponding gutmicrobiota profile are linked to a lower risk of type 2 diabetes, independent of the presence of obesity." *Clin Nutr*. 2020; 39: 524-32.
226. Steen E, Terry BM, Rivera E.J., et al." Impaired insulin and insulin-like growth factor expression and signaling mechanisms in Alzheimer's disease--is this type 3 diabetes?" *J Alzheimers Dis*. 2005; 7: 63-80.

227. Ahmad W. "Overlapped metabolic and therapeutic links between Alzheimer and diabetes." *Mol Neurobiol.*2013; 47: 399-424.
228. de la Monte S.M, Re E, Longato L, et al. "Dysfunctional pro-ceramide, ER stress, and insulin/IGF signaling networks with progression of Alzheimer's disease." *J Alzheimers Dis.* 2012; 30 Suppl 2: S217-29.
229. Querfurth H.W, La Ferla F.M. "Alzheimer's Disease." *N Engl J Med* 2010; 362: 329-4226.
230. Takeuchi M, Yamagishi S. "Possible involvement of advanced glycation end-products (AGEs) in the pathogenesis of Alzheimer's disease." *Curr Pharm Des.* 2008; 14: 973-8.
231. Maillard, L. C. "Action des acides aminés sur les sucres: formation des mélanoïdines par voieméthodique." Compte-rendu de l'Académie des Scienc.1912; 154: 66-8.
232. Rossi J.P.F.C. Combinación de sabores. Ciencia Hoy. 2015; 24: 52-5.
233. Koening R.J, Peterson C.M, Jones R.L, et al. "Correlation of glucose regulation and haemoglobin Alc in diabetes mellitus." *N Engl J Med.* 1976; 295: 417-20.
234. De Christopher L.R. Perspective: "The Paradox in Dietary Advanced Glycation End Products Research-The Source of the Serum and Urinary Advanced Glycation End Products Is the Intestines, Not the Food." *Adv Nutr.* 2017; 8: 679-3.
235. Bains Y, Gugliucci A, Caccavello R. "Advanced glycation endproducts form during ovalbumin digestion in the presence of fructose: Inhibition by chlorogenic acid." *Fitoterapia.* 2017; 120: 1-5.
236. Khaw K.T, Wareham N, Luben R, et al. "Glycated haemoglobin, diabetes and mortality in men in Norfolk cohort of European prospective investigation on cancer and nutrition." *EPIC-Norfolk.* BMJ. 2001; 322: 15-8.
237. González Flecha F.L, Castello P.R, Gagliardino J.J, et al. "La glucosilación no enzimática de proteínas. Mecanismo y papel de la reacción en la diabetes y el envejecimiento." *Ciencia al dia.* 2000; 3: 1-17.
238. Malgorzata T, Hendriks W.H, Wichers H.J, el al. "Immunomodulation by processed animal feed: The role of Maillard reaction products and advanced glycation end products (AGES)." *Front Immunol.* 2018; 9: 2088.

239. Bengmark S. "Advanced glycation and lipoxidation end products amplifiers of inflammation: The role of food." *J Parent Enter Nutr.* 2007; 31: 430-40.
240. Uribarri J, Cai W, Peppa M, et al. "Circulating glycotoxins and dietary advanced glycation endproducts: two links to inflammatory response, oxidative stress and ageing." *J Gerontol.* 2007; 62A: 427-33.
241. Gkogkolou P, Böhm M. "Advanced glycation end products: Key players in skin ageing?" *Dermato-endocrinology.* 2012; 4; 259-70.
242. Voyer LE., Alvarado C. "Reacción de Maillard. Efectos patogénicos." *Medicina* (Buenos Aires). 2019; 79: 137-43.
243. Enzinger C, Fazekas F, Matthews P.M, et al. "Risk factors for progression of brain atrophy in ageing: six-year follow-up of normal subjects." *Neurology.* 2005; 64: 1704-11.
244. Rosenbloom AL, Silverstein J.H, Lezotte DC, et al. "Limited Joint Mobility in Childhood Diabetes Mellitus Indicates Increased Risk for Microvascular Disease." *N Eng J Med.* 1981; 305: 191-4.
245. Voyer L.E. Bruno O. Ibarra R. et al. "Nefropatía diabética en la infancia." Rev Hosp Gral Niños Dr Pedro de Elizalde. 1997; 7: 23.
246. Birlouez-Aragon I, Saavedra G, Tessier FJ, et al. "A diet based on high-heat-treated foods promotes risk factors for diabetes mellitus and cardiovascular diseases." *Am J Clin Nutr.* 2010; 91: 1220-6.
247. Levi B; Werman M.J. "Long-term fructose consumption accelerates glycation and several age-related variables in male rats." *J Nutr.* 1998; 128: 1442.
248. Richard D, Semba R.D, Gebauer S.K., et al. "Dietary Intake of Advanced Glycation End Products Did Not Affect Endothelial Function and Inflammation in Healthy Adults in a Randomized Controlled Trial." *J Nutr.* 2014; 144: 1037-42.
249. Uribarri J, del Castillo M.D, de la Maza M.P., et al. "Dietary advanced glycation end products and their role in health and disease." *Adv Nutr.* 2015; 6: 461-73.
250. Kong Y, Li X, Zheng T., et al. "Glycation of β-lactoglobulin and antiglycation by genistein in different reactive carbonyl model systems." *Food Chem.* 2015; 183: 36-42.
251. Voyer L.E. "Síndromes malformativos. Secuencia de retracción caudal. En: Voyer, Ruvinsky, Cambiano." *Pediatría.* 3ra Ed. 2011; 14.11: 1101. Ed. Journal, Buenos Aires.
252. Smit A.J, Gerrits E.G. "Skin autofluorescence as a measure of advanced glycation endproduct deposition: a novel risk marker in

chronic kidney disease." *Curr Opin Nephrol Hypertens.* 2010; 19: 527-33.

253. Meerwaldt R, Hartog J.W, Graaff R., et al. "Skin autofluorescence, a measure of cumulative metabolic stress and advanced glycation end products, predicts mortality in hemodialysis patients." *J Am Soc* Nephrol. 2005; 16: 3687-93.
254. Gerrits E.G, Lutgers H.L, Smeets G.H.W, et al. "Autofluorescence: A Pronounced Marker of Mortality in Hemodialysis Patients." *Nephron Extra.* 2012; 2: 184–91.
255. Uribarri J, He J.C. "The Low AGE Diet: A Neglected Aspect of Clinical Nephrology." *Nephron.* 2015; 130: 48-53.
256. Dearlove RP, Greenspan P, Hartle D.K. et al. "Inhibition of protein glycation by extracts of culinary herbs and spices." *J Med Food.* 2008; 11: 275-81.
257. Hagen T.M, Liu J.L, Lykkesfeldt J. et al. "Acetyl-L-carnitine and lipo-acid to old rats significantly improves metabolic function while decreasing oxidative stress." *Proc Nat iAcad Sci* USA. 2002; 99: 1870-5.
258. Mizutani K, Ikeda K, Yamory Y. "Resveratrol inhibits AGEs-induced proliferation and collagen synthesis activity in vascular smooth muscle cells from stroke-prone spontaneously hypertensive rats." *Biochem Biophys Res Commun.* 2000; 274: 61-7.
259. Liu Y, He X.Q, Huang X, et al. "Resveratrol protects mouse oocytes from methylglyoxal-induced oxidative damage." *PloSOne.* 2013; 8: e7796.
260. Couppé C, Svensson R.B, Grosset J.F. et al. "Life-long endurance running is associated with reduced glycation and mechanical stress in connective tissue." *Age* Dordrecht: Netherlands, 2014; 36: 9665.
261. Pageon H, Zucchi H, Rousset F. et al. "Skin ageing by glycogen: lessons from the reconstructed skin model." *Clin Chem Lab Med.* 2014; 52: 169-74.
262. Cefalu W.T, Bell-Farrow AD, Wang Z.Q. et al. "Caloric restriction decreases age-dependent accumulation of the glycoxidation products, N epsilon (carboxymethyl) lysine and pentosidine, in the rat skin collagen." *J Gerontol Biol Sci Med Sci.* 1995; 50: B337-41.
263. Grey A.D. "A proposed refinement of the mitochondrial free radical theory of ageing." *Bioessays.* 1997; 19: 161-6.
264. Toda M, Hellwig M, Henle T. et al. "Influence of the Maillard Reaction on the Allergenicity of Food Proteins and the Development of Allergic Inflammation." *Curr Allergy Asthma Rep.* 2019; 19: 4.

265. Teodorowicz M, van Neerven J, Savelkoul H. "Food Processing: The Influence of the Maillard Reaction on Immunogenicity and Allergenicity of Food Proteins." *Nutrients*.2017; 9: 835.
266. Warburg O, Posener K, Negelin E. "Uber den Stoffwechsel der Carcinomzelle." *Biochem Z*. 1924; 152: 319-44.
267. Warburg O. "On the Origin of Cancer Cells." *Science* 1956; 123: 309-14.
268. Gogvadze V, Orrennius S, Zhivotovsky B. "Mitochondria in cancer cells: what is so special about them?" *Trends in Cell Biology*. 2008; 18: 165-73.
269. Margulis L, Bermudes D. "Symbiosis as a mechanism of evolution: Status of cell symbiosis theory." *Symbiosis*. 1985; 1: 101-24.
270. Gray M.W. "Origin and evolution of mitochondrial DNA." *Annu Rev Cell Biol*. 1989; 5: 25-50.
271. Gray M.W. "Mitocondrial Evolution." *Cold Spring Harb Perspect Biol*. 2012; 4: a011403.
272. Gray M.W. "Mosaic nature of the mitochondrial proteome: implications for the origin and evolution of mitochondria." *Proc Natl Acad Sci* USA. 2015; 112: 10133-8.
273. Veltri K.L, Espiritu M, Singh G. "Distinct genomic copy number in mitochondria of different mammalian organs." *J Cell Physiol*.1990; 43: 160-4.
274. Shen J, Gopalakrishnan V, Lee J.E. "Mitochondrial DNA copy number in peripheral blood and melanoma risk." *PLoSOne* 2015; 10: e0131649.
275. Zeviar D.D. Gonzalez M.J, Miranda Massari J.R., et al. "The role of mitochondria in cancer and other chronic diseases." *J Orthomol Med*. 2014; 29: 157-66.
276. Neustadt J, Pieczenik SR. "Medication-induced mitochondrial damage and disease." *Mol Nutr Food* Res. 2008; 52: 78.
277. Kermode-Scott B. "Taking non-aspirin NSAIDs in early pregnancy doubles risk of miscarriage, study shows." *BMJ*. 2011; 343: d5769.
278. SuayLlopis L, Ballester Diaz F. "Revisión de los estudios sobreexposición al aluminio y su relación con la enfermedad de Alzheimer." *Rev Esp Salud Pública*. 2002; 76 Nº 6.
279. Curhan SG, Eavey R, Shargorodsky J, et al. "Analgesic use and the risk of hearing loss in men." *Am J Med*. 2010; 123: 231-7.
280. Voyer L.E, Walther J.C, Bredeston L, et al. "Intoxicación salicílica en Pediatría." Premio Navarro. *Acad Medicina de Buenos Aires*. 1975. Arch Arg Pediatr. 1977; 75: 254-77.

281. Voyer L.E, Pereyra B.A. "Efecto de los salicilatos sobre la gluconeogénesis renal." *Medicina* (Buenos Aires). 1974; 34: 633.
282. Gogvadze V, Zhivotovsky B, Orrenius S. "The Warburg effect and mitochondrial stability in cancer cells." *Mol Aspects Med.* 2010; 31: 60-74.
283. Kidd, PM. "Neurodegeneration from mitochondrial insufficiency: Nutrients, stem cells, growth factors and prospects for brain rebuilding using integrative management." *Alt Med Rev.* 2005; 10: 268-93.
284. González M.J, Miranda Massari J.R, Duconge J, et al. "The bio-energetic theory of carcinogenesis. Med Hypoth." 2012; 79: 433-9.
285. Alarcón-Aguilar A, Maycotte-González P, Cortés-Hernández P, et al. "Dinámica mitocondrial en las enfermedades neurodegenerativas." *Gac Med Mex.* 2019; 155: 276-83.
286. Wallace DC. "A mitochondrial paradigm of metabolic and degenerative diseases, ageing, and cancer: A dawn for evolutionary medicine." *An Rev Genet.* 2005; 39: 359-407.
287. Cohen BH., Gold D.R. "Mitochondrial cytopathy in adults: what we know so far." *Clev Clin J Med.* 2001; 68: 625-6.
288. Cho H, Budhathoki S, Kanehara R. et al. "Association between dietary sugar intake and colorectal adenoma among cancer screening examinees in Japan." *Cancer Sci.* 2020; 111: 3862-72.
289. Gorska-Ciebiada M, Saryusz-Wolska M, Borkowska A. et al. "C-Reactive Protein, Advanced Glycation End Products and Their Receptor in Type 2 Diabetic, Elderly Patients with Mild Cognitive Impairment." *Front Ageing Neurosci.* 2015; 29:7:209.
290. Klement RJ, Kämmerer U. "Is there a role for carbohydrate restriction in the treatment and prevention of cancer?" *Nutr Metab* (Lond). 2011: 26; 8: 75.
291. Zamzami N, Roemer G. "The mitochondrion in apoptosis how Pandora's box opens." *Nat Rev Mol Cel Biol.* 2001; 2: 67-71
292. Michelakis E.D, Webster L, Mackey JR. "Dichloroacetate (DCA) as a potential metabolic-targeting therapy for cancer." *Brit J Cancer.* 2008; 99: 989-94.
293. Zeviar D.D, Gonzalez M.J, Miranda Massari J.R, et al. "The role of mitochondria in cancer and other chronic diseases." *J Orthomo l Med.* 2014; 29: 157-66.
294. González M.J, Miranda Massari J.R, Duconge J, et al. "The bio-energetic theory of carcinogenesis. Med Hypotheses." 2012; 79: 433-9.

295. Davila A.F, Zamorano P. "Mitochondria and the evolutionary roots of cancer." *Phys Biol.* 2013; 10: 026008.
296. Klement R.J, Kämmerer U. "Is there a role for carbohydrate restriction in the treatment and prevention of cancer?" *Nutr Metab* (Lond). 2011; 8: 75.
297. Graham N.A, Tahmasian M, Kohli B, et al. "Glucose deprivation activates a metabolic and signaling amplification loop leading to cell death." *Mol Syst Biol.* 2012; 8: 589.
298. Quade B.N, Parker M.D, Occhipinti R. "The therapeutic importance of acid-base balance." Biochem Pharmacol. 2021; 183: 114278.
299. Minich D, Bland J. "Acid-alkaline balance: Role in chronic disease and detoxification." *Alt Therap Health Med.* 2007; 13, 62-5.
300. Veech, R. "The therapeutic implications of ketone bodies: the effects of ketone bodies in pathological conditions: ketosis, ketogenic diet, redox states, insulin resistance and mitochondrial metabolism." Prostaglandins Leukot Essent Fatty Acids. 2004; 70: 309-28
301. Vantallie T.B, Nufert T.H. "Ketones: metabolism's ugly duckling." *Nutr Rev.* 2003, 61, 327-41.
302. Maurer G.D, Brucker D.P, Bâhr O. et al." Differential utilization of ketone bodies by neurons and glioma cell lines: a rationale for ketogenic diet as experimental glioma therapy." *BMC Cancer.* 2011; 11: 315.
303. Davila A.F, Zamorano P. "Mitochondria and the evolutionary roots of cancer." *Phys Biol.* 2013; 10: 026008.
304. Gundamaraju R, Lu W, Manikam R. "Revisiting Mitochondria Scored Cancer Progression and Metastasis." *Cancers* (Basel). 2021; 13: 432.
305. Minich D, Bland J. "Acid-alkaline balance: Role in chronic disease and detoxification." *Alt Therap Health Med.* 2007; 13, 62-5.
306. Zhou W, Mukherjee P, Kiebish M.A. et al. "The calorically restricted ketogenic diet, an effective alternative therapy for malignant brain cancer." *Nutr Metab.* 2007; 4: 1-15.
307. Nicolson G, Ash M.E. "Membrane Lipid Replacement for chronic illnesses, ageing and cancer using oral glycerolphospholipid formulations with fructooligosaccharides to restore phospholipid function in cellular membranes, organelles, cells and tissues." *BiochBioph Acta* (BBA) - Biomem. 2017; 1869: 1704-24.

308. Poff A.M, Ari C Seyfried T.N, D'Agostino D.P. et al. "The ketogenic diet and hyperbaric oxygen prolong survival in mice with systemic metastatic cancer." *PLoS One*. 2013: 8: e65522.
309. Watson W.H, Cai J, Jones D.P. Diet and apoptosis. Annu Rev Nut. 2000; 29: 485-05.
310. Macfarlane C.M. "Sublethal oxygen deficiency—the primary cause of cancer." *Medical Hypotheses*. 2000; 54: 323–5.
311. Gill A.L, Bell C.N.A. "Hyperbaric oxygen: its uses, mechanisms of action and outcomes." QJM. 2004; 97: 385-95.
312. Nicolson G.L. "Lipid replacement as an adjunct to therapy for chronic fatigue, anti-ageing and restoration of mitochondrial function." *J Am Nutraceut Assoc*. 2003; 6: 22-8.
313. Nicolson G.L, Ellithorpe R. "Lipid replacement and antioxidant nutritional therapy for restoring mitochondrial function and reducing fatigue in chronic fatigue syndrome and other fatiguing illnesses." *J ChrFatig Synd*. 2006; 13: 57-68
314. Biyikli N.K, Gokce I, Cakalagoglu F. et al. "The coexistence of membranoproliferative glomerulonephritis type I and coeliac disease: a case report." *Pediatr Nephrol*. 2009; 24: 1247-50.
315. Hadjivassilio M, Sanders DA, Grunewald R.A, et al. "Gluten sensitivity: from gut to brain." *Lancet* Neurol. 2010; 9: 318–30.
316. Versino M, Biagi F, Bianchi P.I, et al. "Gluten sensitivity and the CNS: diagnosis and treatment." Lancet Neurol. 2010; 9: 653.
317. Mansueto P, Seidita A, D'Alcamo A. et al. "Non-Coeliac gluten sensitivity: litreature review." *3* 2014; 33: 39-54.
318. Mataix J. "Síndromes de maldigestión y malabsorción." En: *Nutrición y Alimentación Humana. Cap*. 38. 979-1005. Ed. Ergón. 2002.
319. Vazquez-Roque MI1, Camilleri M, Smyrk T. et al. "A controlled trial of gluten-free diet in patients with irritable bowel syndrome-diarrhoea: effects on bowel frequency and intestinal function." *Gastroenterol*.2013; 144: 903-11. e3.
320. Uranga J.A, Martínez V, Abalo R. "Mast Cell Regulation and Irritable Bowel Syndrome: Effects of Food Components with Potential Nutraceutical Use." *Molecules*. 2020; 25: 4314.
321. Bellini M, Tomarelli, S, Mumolo M.G. et al. "Low Fermentable Oligo- Di- and Mono-Saccharides and Polyols (FODMAPs) or Gluten Free Diet: What Is Best for Irritable Bowel Syndrome?" *Nutrients*. 2020; 12: 3368.

322. Paray B.A, Albeshr M.F, Jan A.T. et al. “Leaky Gut and Autoimmunity: An Intricate Balance in Individuals Health and the Diseased State.” *Int J Mol Sci*. 2020; 21: 9770.
323. Mumolo M.G, Rettura F, Melissari S. et al. “Is Gluten the Only Culprit for Non-Coeliac Gluten/Wheat Sensitivity?” *Nutrients*. 2020; 12: 3785.
324. Barbaro M.R, Cremon C, Wrona D. et al. “Non-Coeliac Gluten Sensitivity in the Context of Functional Gastrointestinal Disorders.” *Nutrients*. 2020; 12: 3735.
325. Volta U, Caio G, Stanghellini V. et al. “The Changing Clinical Profil of Coeliac Disease BMC Gastroenterol.” 2014; 14: 194.
326. Cordain L, Toohey L, Smith M.J. et al. “Modulation of immune function by dietary lectins in rheumatoid arthritis.” *Br J Nutr*. 2000; 83: 207-17.
327. Makhlouf S, Messelmani M, Zaouali J. et al. “Cognitive impairment in coeliac disease and non-coeliac gluten sensitivity: review of literature on the main cognitive impairments, the imaging and the effect of gluten-free diet.” *Acta Neurol Belg*. 2018; 118: 21-7.
328. Lerner A, Benzvi C. “Let Food Be Thy Medicine”: Gluten and Potential Role in Neurodegeneration. Cells. 2021;10: 756.
329. Llorens S, Nava E, Muñoz-López M. et al. “Neurological Symptoms of COVID-19: The Zonulin Hypothesis.” *Front Immunol*. 2021; 12: 665300.
330. Sharma L, Riva A. “Intestinal Barrier Function in Health and Disease-Any role of SARS-CoV-2?” *Microorganisms*. 2020; 8: 1744.
331. Genuis SJ, Bouchard T.P. “Celiac disease presenting as autism.” *J Child Neurol*. 2010; 25: 114-19.
332. Pennesi C.M, Klein L.C. “Effectiveness of the gluten-free, casein-free diet for children diagnosed with autism spectrum disorder: based on parental report.” *Nutr Neurosci*. 2012; 15: 85-91.
333. Cekici H, Sanlier N. “Current nutritional approaches in managing autism spectrum disorder: A review.” *Nutr Neurosc*. 2019; 22: 145-55.
334. Samsel, A, Seneff, S. “Glyphosate’s Suppression of Cytochrome P450 Enzymes and Amino Acid Biosynthesis by the Gut Microbiome: Pathways to Modern Diseases.” *Entropy* 2013; 15: 1416-63.
335. Álvarez Vidal L, Iglesias Cid I. Asignatura Fundamentos de Alimentación y Nutrición. Cap. 1. Productos alimentarios. Aspectos negativos de las leguminosas. Pg. 14. Maestría de Nutrición y

Dietética. Univ. Europea Miguel de Cervantes. 2013. Mataix Verdú D.J. Recomendaciones nutricionales y alimentarias. En: Nutrición y Alimentación Humana. Cap 10. Ed. Ergón

336. Vojdani A, Afar D, Vojdani E. "Reaction of Lectin-Specific Antibody with Human Tissue: Possible Contributions to Autoimmunity." *J Immunol Res*. 2020; 2020:1438957.
337. Jonsson T, Olsson S, Wu Xiao C, et al. "Agrarian diet and diseases of affluence. Do evolutionary novel dietary lectins cause leptin resistance?" *BMC Endocrine Disorders*. 2005; 5: 10.
338. Vekua A, Lordkipanidze D, Rightmire GP, et al. "A new skull of early *Homo* from Dmanisi, Georgia." *Science*. 2002; 297: 85-9.
339. Green R.E. "A draft sequence of the neandertal genome." *Science*. 2010; 328: 710-22.340.
341. Krause J, Fu Q, Good J.M, et al. "The complete mitochondrial DNA genome of an unknown hominin from southern Siberia." *Nature*. 2010; 464: 894-97.
342. Aguirre P. "Del gramillon al aspartamo. Las transiciones alimentarias en el tiempo de la especie." *Boletín Techint* N° 306 Mayo-Junio 2001.
343. Escudero P. "Las vitaminas." (Tercera parte). En: *Alimentación*. Pg. 116. Librería Hachette S.A. Buenos Aires. 1934.
344. Escudero P. "Alimentación y composición química de los tejidos". En: *Alimentación*. Segunda parte. Influencia de la alimentación sobre la duración de la vida. 134. Librería Hachette S.A. Buenos Aires. 1934.
345. Organización Panamericana de la Salud, Organización Mundial de la Salud. Alimentos y Bebidas Ultraprocesados En América Latina. 2019.
346. Monteiro C.A, Levy R.B, Claro R.M. et al. "A new classification of foods based on the extent and purpose of their processing." *Cad Saude Publica*. 2010; 26: 2039-49.
347. Martínez Steele E, Khandpur N, Da Costa Louzada M. et al. Association between dietary contribution of ultra-processed foods and urinary concentrations of phthalates and bisphenol in a nationally representative sample of the US population aged 6 years and older." PLoS One. 2020; 15: 1-21.
348. Rancière F, Lyons J.G, Loh V.H. et al. "Bisphenol A and the risk of cardiometabolic disorders: a systematic review with meta-analysis of the epidemiological evidence." *Environ Health*. 2015; 31; 14:46.
349. Justich P.R. "¿Medicina basada en el mercado o medicina basada en el paciente?" *Arch Argent Pediatr*. 2015; 113: 146-53.

350. Voyer L.E. Medio interno. "Fisiología, patología y tratamiento de los líquidos orgánicos." *Ed. Journal*. Buenos Aires. 2017.
351. Bricker N.S, Bourgoingnie J.J, Webwe H. "The renal response to progressive nephron loss." In Brenner BM, Rector FC. *The Kidney*. Chapter 18. WB. Saunders Comp. 1976. Phil.
352. Segunda Encuesta Nacional de Factores de Riesgo 2005-2009. Enfermedades no transmisibles. Ministerio Nacional de Salud. Presidencia de la Nación. República Argentina.
353. Mataix Verdú J, Pérez Llamas F. "Alimentos del futuro: Alimentos funcionales y transgénicos." En: *Nutrición y Alimentación humana*. 2ª ed.Cap.19. Ed Argón. Madrid. 2009. 4.
354. Alzamora S.M, Salvatori D, Tapia SM. et al. "Novel functional foods from vegetable matrices impregnated with biologically active compounds." *J Food Eng*. 2005; 67:205–1
355. Niva M. "All foods affect health: understandings of functional foods and healthy eating among health-oriented Finns." *Appetite*. 2007; 48:384-93
356. Castellari E, Ricci E.C, Stranieri S. "Relationships Between Health and Environmental Information on the Willingness to Pay for Functional Foods: The Case of a New Aloe Vera Based Product." *Nutrients*. 2019; 11: 2781
357. Ursashi C.Ş, Perţa-Crişan S, Munteanu FD. "Strategies to Improve Meat Products" *Quality Foods*. 2020; 9: 1883
358. Clifford T, Howatson G, West D.J. et al. "The potential benefits of red beetroot supplementation in health and disease." *Nutrients*. 2015; 7: 2801-22.
359. Domínguez R, Cuenca E, Maté-Muñoz J.L. et al. "Effect of beetroot supplementation on cardiorespiratory endurance in athletes." *A systemic review*. Nutrients 2017; 9: 43
360. Lu S.C. "Glutathione synthesis." *Biochim Biophys Acta*. 2013; 1830: 3143-53.
361. Minich D.M, Brown B.I. "A Review of Dietary (Phyto)Nutrients for Glutathione Support." *Nutrients*. 2019; 11: 2073
362. Manach C, Scalbert A, Morand C. et al. "Polyphenols: food sources and bioavailability." *Am J Clin Nutr*. 2004; 79: 727-47
363. Brüll V, Burak C, Stoffel-Wagner B. et al. "Effects of a quercetin-rich onion skin extract on 24 h ambulatory blood pressure and endothelial function in weight gain-to-obese patients with pre-hypertension: a randomised double-blinded placebo-controlled cross-over trial." *Br J Nutr*. 2015; 114: 1263-77

364. Edwards R.L, Lyon T, Litwin S.E.et al. "Quercetin reduces blood pressure in hypertensive subjects." *J Nutr*. 2007; 137: 2405-11.
365. Kawai Y, Nishikawa T, Shiba Y. et al. "Macrophage as a target of quercetin glucuronides in human atherosclerotic arteries: implication in the anti-atherosclerotic mechanism of dietary flavonoids." *J Biol Chem*. 2008; 283: 9424-34.
366. Menendez C, Dueñas M, Galindo P, et al. "Vascular deconjugation of quercetin glucuronide: The flavonoid paradox revealed?" *Mol Nutr Food Res*. 2011; 55: 1780-90
367. Batiha GE, Beshbishy A.M, Ikram M. et al. "The Pharmacological Activity, Biochemical Properties, and Pharmacokinetics of the Major Natural Polyphenolic Flavonoid: Quercetin. Foods." 2020; 9: 374.
368. Soeur J, Eilstein J, Lereaux G. et al. "Skin resistance to oxidative stress induced by resveratrol: from Nrf2 activation to GSH biosynthesis." *Free Radic Biol Med*. 2015; 78: 213-23
369. Kwon S.H, Park K.C. "Antioxidants as an Epidermal Stem Cell Activator." *Antioxidants* (Basel). 2020; 9: 958.
370. Duarte J, Pérez-Vizcaíno F. "Cardiovascular protection by flavonoids. Pharmacokinetic mystery." *Ars Pharm*. 2015; 56: 193-200.
371. Zenebe W, Pechánová O, Bernátová I. "Protective effects of red wine polyphenolic compounds on the cardiovascular system." *Exp Clin Cardiol*. 2001; 6: 153-8
372. Szmitko P.E, Vermam S. Cardiology patient pages. "Red wine and your health." Circulation. 2005; 111: e10-1.
373. Toyokuni S, Okamoto K, Yodoi J, et al. "Persistent oxidative stress in cancer." *FEBS let*. 1995; 16: 1-3.
374. Hirano T, Fukuoka K, Oka K. et al. "Antiproliferative activity of mammalian lignan derivatives against the human breast carcinoma cell line, ZR-75-1." *J Cancer Res Clin Oncol*.2003; 29: 569-76
375. Thompson L.U. "Experimental studies on lignans and cancer." *Metabolism*. 1998; 12: 691-705
376. Fabiani R, De Bartolomeo A, Rosignoli P. et al. "Virgin Oil Phenols inhibit Proliferation of Human Promyelocytic Leukemia Cells (HL60) by inducing Apoptosis and Differentiation." *J Nutr*. 2006; 136: 614-19
377. Fortes C, Forastiere F, Farchi S. et al. "The protective effect of the Mediterranean diet on lung cancer." *Nutr Cancer*. 2003; 46: 30-7.

378. Higuera Campo J. "Los compuesos fenólicos en el aceite de oliva/hojas oliva: propiedades beneficiosas." Julio 2017. Universidad Cantábrica.
379. Stahl W, Sies H. "Uptake of lycopene and its geometrical isomers is greater from heat processed than from unprocessed tomato juice in humans." J Nutr 1992; 122: 2161-6.
380. Gartner C, Stahl W, Sies H. "Lycopene is more bioavailable from tomato paste than from fresh tomatoes." *Am J Clin Nutr*. 1997; 66:116-22.
381. Maruyama C, Imamura K, Oshima S, et al. "Effects of tomato juice consumption on plasma and lipoprotein carotenoid concentrations and the susceptibility of low-density lipoprotein to oxidative modification." *J Nutr Sci Vitaminol* (Tokyo). 2001; 47: 213-21
382. Nkondjock A, Ghasirian P, Johnson KC, et al. Canadian Cancer Registries Epidemiology Research Group. "Dietary intake of lycopene is associated with reduced pancreatic cancer risk." *J Nutr.*2005; 135: 592-7.
383. Cruz Bojórquez R.M, González Gallego J, Sánchez Collado P. Revisión. "Propiedades funcionales y beneficios para la salud del licopeno." *NutrHosp.*2013; 28: 6-15
384. Paran E, Peter, W, Aalt Bast. "Tomato Extract for Hypertension?" Editorial to "The Effects of Natural Antioxidants from Tomato Extract in Treated but Uncontrolled Hypertensive Patients" *Cardiovascular Drugs and Therapy*. 2009; 23: 107-8
385. Li Y, Go V.L, Sarkar F.H. "The Role of Nutraceuticals in Pancreatic Cancer Prevention and Therapy: Targeting Cellular Signaling, Micro RNAs and Epigenome." *Pancreas.*2015; 44: 1-10
386. Jurenka, J.S. "Anti-inflammatory properties of curcumin, a major constituent of curcuma longa: a review of preclinical and clinical research" *Alter Med Rev*. 2009; 14: 141-53.
387. Schaffer M, Schaffer P.M, Bar-Sela G. "An update on Curcuma as a functional food in the control of cancer and inflammation." *Curr Opin Clin Nutr Metab Care*. 2015; 18: 605-11
388. Lao C.D, Ruffin M.T, Normolle D. et al. "Safety & Dosage Review: Curcumin. Dose escalation of a curcuminoid formulation." *Complement Altern Med*. 2006; 6: 10.
389. Kanai M, Imaizumi A, Otsuka Y. et al. "Dose-escalation and Pharmacokinetic Study of Nanoparticle Curcumin, a Potential Anticancer Agent with Improved Bioavailability, in Healthy Human Volunteers." *Cancer Chemother Pharmacol*. 2012; 69: 65

390. Shoba G, Joy D, Joseph T. et al. "Influence of Piperine on the Pharmacokinetics of Curcumin in Animals and Human Volunteers" *Planta Med.* 1998; 64: 353-6.
391. Chen Y, Lu Y, Lee R.J. et al. "Nano encapsulated curcumin its potential for biomedical applications. Int J Nanomedicine" 2020; 15: 3099-3120
392. Srinivasan K. "Black pepper and its pungent principle-piperine: a review of diverse physiological effects." *Crit Rev Food Sci Nutr.* 2007; 47: 735-48
393. Shao B, Cui C, Ji H. et al. "Enhanced oral bioavailability of piperine by self-emulsifying drug delivery systems: in vitro, in vivo and in situ intestinal permeability studies." *Drug Deliv.* 2015; 22: 740-7.
394. Ren T, Zuo Z. "Role of piperine in CNS diseases: pharmacodynamics, pharmacokinetics and drug interactions." *Expert Opin Drug Metab Toxicol.* 2019; 15: 849-67
395. Bourassa P, Kanankis C.D, Tarantilis M.G. et al. "Resveratrol, genistein and curcumin bind bovine serum albumin." *J Phys Chem B.* 2010; 114: 3348-54.
396. Feng J, Wu S, Wang H. et al. "Improved bioavailability of curcumin in ovalbumin-dextran nanogel prepared by Maillard reaction." *J Funct Foods.* 2016; 27: 55-68
397. Ghayour N, Hosseini S.M.H, Esckandari M.H. et al. "Nanoencapsulated of quercetin and curcumin in casein based delivery systems." *Food Hydrocolloids.* 2019; 87: 394-403
398. Panahi Y, Hosseini M.S, Khalili N. et al. "Antioxidant and anti-inflammatory effects of curcuminoid-piperine combination in subjects with metabolic syndrome: A randomized controlled trial and an updated meta-analysis." *Clin Nutr.* 2015; 34: 1101-8
399. Tasleem F, Azhar I, Ali S.N. et al. "Analgesic and anti-inflammatory activities of Piper nigrum L. Asian Pac" *J Trop Med.* 2014; 7S1: S461-8.
400. Kuptniratsaikul V, Thanakhumtorn S, Chinswangwatanakul P. et al. "Efficacy and safety of Curcuma domestica extracts in patients with knee osteoarthritis." *Int J Mol Med.* 2010; 25: 729-34
401. Daily J.W, Yang M, Park S. "Efficacy of Turmeric Extracts and Curcumin for Alleviating the Symptoms of Joint Arthritis: A Systematic Review and Meta-Analysis of Randomized Clinical Trials." *J Med Food.*2016; 19: 717-29.

402. Henrotin Y, Clutterbuck A.L, Allaway D. et al. "Biological actions of curcumin on articular chondrocytes." *Osteoarthr Cartil.* 2010; 18: 141-9
403. Lim G.P, Chu T, Yang F. et al." The curry spice curcumin reduces oxidative damage and amyloid pathology in an Alzheimer transgenic mouse." *J Neurosci.* 2001; 21: 8370-77
404. Wajab A.N.A, Lajis N.H, Abas F. et al. "Mechanism of Anti-Cancer Activity of Curcumin on Androgen-Dependent and Androgen-Independent Prostate Cancer." *Nutrients.*2020; 12: 679
405. Kunnumakkara A.B, Bordoloi, D, Harsha Ch. et al. "Curcumin Mediates Anticancer Effects by Modulating Multiple Cell Signaling Pathways." *Clin Sci.* 2017; 131: 1781-99
406. Pescosolido N, Giannotti R, Plateroti A.M. et al. "Curcumin: terapeutical potential in ophtalmology." *Planta Med.* 2014; 80: 249-54
407. Panaro M.A, Corrado A, Benameur T. et al. "Therapeutic Effects of Curcumin, the Anti-inflammatory Agent, Against Neurodegenerative, Cardiovascular, Pulmonary, Metabolic, Autoimmune and Neoplastic Diseases." *Int J Biochem Cell Biol.* 2009; 41: 40-59.
409. Stohs S.J, Chen O, Ray S.D. et al. "Highly Bioavailable Forms of Curcumin and Promising Avenues for Curcumin-Based Research and Application: A Review." *Molecules* 2020; 25: 1397.
410. Ahmad R.S, Hussain M.B, Sultan M.T. et al. "Biochemistry, Safety, Pharmacological Activities, and Clinical Applications of Turmeric: A Mechanistic Review." *Evid Based Complement Alternat Med.* 2020; 2020: 7656919.
411. Shehzad A, Ha T, Subhan F. et al. "New mechanisms and the anti-inflammatory role of curcumin in obesity and obesity related metabolic diseases." *Eur J Med.* 2011; 50: 151-61.
412. Shao W, Yu Z, Chiang Y, et al. "Curcumin prevents high fat diet induced insulin resistance and obesity via attenuating lipogenesis in liver and inflammatory pathway in adipocytes." *PLoS ONE.* 2012; 7e28784.
413. Gómez-Téllez A, Sierra-Puente D, Muñoz-Gómez R. et al. "Effects of a Low-Dose Spirulina/Turmeric Supplement on Cardiometabolic and Antioxidant Markers of Patients With Abdominal Obesity."
Front Nutr. 2020; 7: 65
414. Nabila N, Suada N.K, Denis D. et al. "Antiviral Action of Curcumin Encapsulated in Nanoemulsion against Four Serotypes of Dengue Virus." *Pharm Nanotechnol.* 2020; 8: 54-62

415. Thimulappa R.K, Mudnakudu-Nagaraju K.K, Shivamallu C. et al. "Antiviral and immunomodulatory activity of curcumin: A case for prophylactic therapy for COVID-19." Heliyon 2021; 7: e06350.
416. Benzie I.F.F. *The amazing and mighty ginger. Herbal Medicine. Biomolecular and Clinical Aspects*. 2nd. Ed.2011.Chapter X. Wachtel-Galor S. Ed. Taylor and Francis. Boca Ratón.
417. Young H.Y, Luo Y.L, Cheng H.Y, et al. "Analgesic and anti-inflammatory activities of [6]- gingerol." *J Ethnopharmacol*. 2005; 96: 207-10.
418. Alizadeh-Navaeis R, Rovzbeeh F, Saravi M. et al. "Investigation of the effect of ginger on the lipid levels. A doubled blind controlled clinical trial." *Saudi Med J*. 2005; 29: 128-4.
419. Vimala S, Norhanom A.W, Yadav M. "Anti-tumour promoting activity in Malaysian ginger rhizobia used in traditional medicine." *Br J Canc*. 1999; 80: 110-6.
420. Prakash U.N.S, Srinivasan K. "Beneficial influence of dietary spices on the ultrastructure and fluidity of the intestinal brush border in rats." *Br J Nutr*. 2010; 24: 1-9.
421. Kieliszek M, Edris A, Kot A.M. "Biological Activity of Sme Aromatic Plants and Their Metabolites, with an Emphasis on Health-Promoting Properties." *Molecules*. 2020; 25: 2478.
422. Gismondi A, Serio M, Canuti L. et al. "Biochemical, antioxidant and antineoplastic properties of Italian saffron (*Crocus sativus* L.)." *Am J Plant Sci*. 2012; 3: 157-380.
423. Nasiri Z, Sameni H.R, Vakili A, et al. "Dietary saffron reduced the blood pressure and prevented remodeling of the aorta in L-NAME-induced hypertensive rats." *Iran J Basic Med Sci*. 2015; 18: 1143-6.
424. Kim Y. "Folic acid fortification and supplementation. Good for some but not so good for others." *Nutr Rev*. 2007; 65: 504-11.
425. Bassaganya-Riera J, Hontecillas R, Horne W.T. et al. "Conjugated linoleic acid modulates immune responses in patients with mild to moderately active Crohn's disease." *Clin Nutr*.2012; 31: 721-27.
426. Tricons S, Burdge G.C, Kew S. et al. "Opposing effects of cis-9 trans-11 and trans-10 cis-12 conjugated linoleic acid on blood lipids in healthy humans." *Am J Clin Nutr*. 2004; 80: 614-20
427. Lee Y. "Isomer specificity of conjugated linoleic acid (CLA): 9E, 11E-CLA." *Nutr Res Pract*. 2008; 2: 326-30.
428. Brown J.M, Boysen M.S, Jensen S.S. et al. "Isomer-specific regulation of metabolism and PRAR gamma signaling by CLA in human preadipocytes." *J Lipid Res*. 2003; 44: 1287-300.

429. Whigham L.D, Watras A.C, Schoeller D.A. "Efficacy of conjugated linoleic acid reducing fat mass: a meta-analysis in humans." *Am J Clin Nutr*. 2007; 85: 1203-11.
430. Den Hartigh L.J. "Conjugated Linoleic Acid Effects on Cancer, Obesity, and Atherosclerosis: A Review of Pre-Clinical and Human Trials with Current Perspectives." *Nutrients*. 2019; 11: 370.
431. Basak S, Asim K. Duttaroy A.K. "Conjugated Linoleic Acid and Its Beneficial Effects in Obesity, Cardiovascular Disease and Cancer." *Nutrients*. 2020; 12: 1913.
432. Mattson M.P, Wan R. "Beneficial effects of intermittent fasting and caloric restriction on the cardiovascular and cerebrovascular systems." *J Nutr Biochem*. 2005;16:129-37.
433. Spindler S.R. "Rapid and reversible induction of the longevity, anticancer and genomic effects of caloric restriction." *Mech Ageing Dev*. 2005;126: 960-6.
434. Burne J. "Can fasting for two days each week stop dementia?" *The Daily Mail*. 2012; February 27.
435. Stallknecht B, Dela F, Helge J.W. "Are blood flow and lipolysis in subcutaneous adipose tissue influenced by contractions in adjacent muscles in humans?" *Am J Physiol-Endocrinol and Metab*. 2007; 292; E394-9.
436. Kennedy D, Jäger R, Mosser D.D, et al. "Regulation of apoptosis by heat shock proteins." IUBMB Life. 2014; 66: 327-38.
437. Madrigal-Matut J, López-Franco O, Blanco-Colio L.M, y col. "Las proteínas de choque térmico (heat shock proteins) como potenciales dianas terapéuticas en aterosclerosis." *Clín Invest Arterioscl*. 2009; 21: 163-72.
438. Ovelgönne J.H, Koninkx J.F, Pusztai A, et al. "Decreased levels of heat shock proteins in gut epithelial cells after exposure to plant lectins." *Gut*. 2000; 46: 679-87.
439. Kabakov A, Yakimova A, Matchuk O. "Molecular Chaperones in Cancer Stem Cells: Determinants of Stemness and Potential Targets for Antitumor Therapy." *Cells*. 2020; 9: 892
440. Schmitt E, Gehrmann M, Brunet M, et al. "Intracellular and extracellular functions of heat shock proteins: repercussions in cancer therapy." *J Leukoc Biol*. 2007; 81: 15-27.
441. Chebotareva N, Bobkova I, Shilov E. "Heat shock proteins and kidney disease: perspectives of HSP therapy." Cell Stress Chaperones. 2017; 22: 319-43.
442. Mercola. "Mouth breathing during exercise may increase your risk for asthma and cardiac problems." Natural Health Website. 2013.

INDEX